the living diet
A Christian Journey to Joyful Eating

Martha Tatarnic

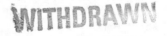

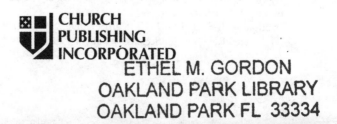
CHURCH
PUBLISHING
INCORPORATED

Dedicated to
St. David, Orillia
&
St. George's, St. Catharines

For a book study guide to accompany *The Living Diet*, go to *www.marthatatarnic.ca* or *https://www.churchpublishing.org/livingdiet*

Church Publishing
19 East 34th Street
New York, NY 10016
www.churchpublishing.org

Cover design by Paul Soupiset
Typeset by Rose Design

Library of Congress Cataloging-in-Publication Data

Names: Tatarnic, Martha, author.
Title: The living diet : a Christian journey to joyful eating / Martha Tatarnic.
Description: New York, NY : Church Publishing, [2019] | Includes bibliographic references.
Identifiers: LCCN 2018055701| ISBN 9781640651487 (pbk.) | ISBN 9781640651494 (ebk.)
Subjects: LCSH: Food—Religious aspects—Christianity. | Nutrition—Religious aspects—Christianity.
Classification: LCC BR115.N87 T38 2019 | DDC 248.4—dc23
LC record available at https://lccn.loc.gov/2018055701

Contents

Introduction

We have an eating disorder. This struggle around how we feed and see our bodies plays out in a variety of ways, and contrary to the stereotypes, it is not confined to a particular age group or gender or to those who are especially obsessed with their appearance. Some of us desperately need to be thinner for health reasons. Most people believe, whether they really need to lose weight or not, that their lives would be better with fewer pounds. Some of us eat to protect or comfort ourselves. Many of us either eat mindlessly or obsessively, stuffing our faces on the run or counting every calorie and carb going into our mouths. Very young children, the middle-aged, seniors, and everyone in between, learn that indulging in food can be a means of filling a void, or that restricting food intake can be a way of asserting power. We are masters at finding and fretting over every perceived imperfection in our own bodies, even as we idolize the "perfect" bodies of the celebrities so glossily depicted in the media.

We are dissatisfied with our bodies, and our dissatisfaction turns into desperation, and our desperation turns into an obsession with food.

I struggled with an eating disorder. On the surface, I was trying to look the way I was taught to look by the culture around me. In a deeper sense, though, I was doing something much more damaging. I was embedding my deepest insecurities into the size of my waistline and believing that my feelings of alienation and despair could be forever lifted if I could just master my relationship with food and bring my body under control.

I was fed and coddled in this belief by a dense fog of media messages, learned eating patterns, cultural norms around dieting, and a nattering and nonstop verbal obsession around bodies—my body, your body, our bodies, celebrity bodies, athletic bodies. All of which taught me that the disgust, frustration, fear, and disappointment I felt about the food I ate and the way my body looked were entirely normal.

Vast amounts of money are channeled into telling us that the secret to health and weight loss can be unlocked . . . if we purchase the right product or adopt the magic discipline. Yet collectively we are getting neither thinner nor happier. We have a big, desperate problem, as big as the excess pounds we carry—both real and imagined—and all of the junk food and junk diets and junk body messages that we keep devouring in between. It isn't just that we are receiving bad teaching about food and bodies. We are also receiving bad *theology* about food and bodies.

Theology—talk about God—gives us language for who we are and what our lives are for. Bad theology makes it commonplace to talk as if food choices are only about me, as if eating is a merely individual act, as if my own pleasure is the ultimate good, even as I am taught that my body is a problem to be solved, or worse, a war to be won.

I am a priest, which means that I regularly have the opportunity to preach to my flock. That being said, I try to guard against "preachiness." At no point have I found that my self-righteous dispensing of advice has been an effective tool in facilitating transformation for others. I think of one particularly long stint on my high horse after successfully getting my baby daughter to sleep through the night after five sleepless months. I liberally preached to all of my new parent friends about my technique, assuring them that I had unlocked the secret to better sleep for them and their babies. None of them was helped by my "expertise," and I was humbled two years later when I discovered that nothing that I had previously done worked with my second child.

This book, then, isn't written from any high horse. After decades of obsessing about food and my body, I did experience healing. But let me be clear. I have never successfully lost weight on a diet. When I have cravings, I usually indulge them. I don't understand anything about gluten and whether or not we should be consuming it. I eat cake, and I enjoy it. This is not a dieting book or even a spiritual companion to your own weight loss program. This is not another part of the wave of internet faith teachers who tell you that God wants you to look after your body as a way of honoring God. I am not going to teach you how to pray instead of eat chips.

What I do have to offer is a rich collection of stories—some of them mine, many of them from the wisdom handed down through the Judeo-Christian faith. I have experience in how these stories allowed me to go from obsessing about food and my body to embrace joyful eating. I was a church-going Christian the whole time my desperation to lose weight was at its peak. It never occurred to me that my faith might have something to say about how I was eating and what I thought about my body. At best, I thought the Christian faith was silent on the matter; at worst, I would have subscribed to a vague notion that God was disappointed with my body too.

I was wrong. Jesus doesn't show us the way to drop pounds or lose inches. He also, thankfully, doesn't point us to a God who wishes we were thinner. The gospel he proclaimed is, however, concerned with the healing and health of our bodies.

But Jesus insists on a different framework. Bad theology teaches that health and healing are just about me. Jesus's gospel teaches that we can learn to honor and appreciate our bodies and our lives when we understand that our bodies and lives are in relationship with other bodies and lives around us.

Amazingly, in upending the bad teaching we have been given about our relationship with food, we might find that we are not just spiritually healthier, but physically as well.

All of the diet plans we could ever need or want are already available to us, teaching us to count calories or eliminate food groups or sign up for the right plan or product. None of them seems to make us any less desperate about food or any less dissatisfied with our bodies. It's time to reclaim the original meaning and intent of the word "diet." "Diet" is a word which comes from the Latin word *diaeta* (or the Greek *diatia*). It literally means "way of life" or "manner of living."

I call this book *The Living Diet* because through the teachings and model of Jesus, we are invited to see hunger, our bodies, and the way that we eat in an entirely different way. This way, this diet, allows us to break out of our own individual spheres of self-concern and into relationship, which is the truest identity of our bodily existence, and which is reaffirmed every time we put food into our mouths. This diet addresses our real eating disorder—our collective eating disorder—an eating disorder that has left us with desperation and dissatisfaction as the norms for how we eat and what we see when we look in the mirror. This diet invites each of us, all of us, to discover the real joy of eating and the true gift of living this bodily existence.

part

1

Disorder

The Dangling Carrot

When I was nine years old, my brother bought a copy of *The Guinness Book of World Records*. I looked nervously at the picture of the Fattest Woman in the World. It was her thighs that captured my eye—roll upon roll of excess weight. Later, in the privacy of my own bedroom, I compared the picture to my own thighs. Laying the book carefully on the floor, I assumed a squatting position, noting with embarrassment the large amount of flab that bulged out along the inner side of my leg. I looked back and forth between what seemed like an enormous amount of flesh on my own thighs and the picture in *Guinness*, wondering if my thighs were as big as the Fattest Woman in the World's.

Looking through the actual photographic record of my nine-year-old self, I now recognize an astonishing thing: *I was not overweight.* There is no picture from my well-documented childhood that even begins to suggest the descriptions I assumed for myself—pudgy, chunky, bigger—whether they came from the words of others, or from my own imagination. But, at nine years old, I was already talking about dieting, already feeling guilty when I ate sweets, already envious of my skinny friends, already holding in my stomach, avoiding that squatting position specifically, and hoping that nobody would notice the many stray rolls that I saw disfiguring my body. Maybe if I wore baggy enough clothes and held my stomach at a certain angle, I could fool people into not seeing the extra flesh that was so obvious to me.

Did I mention that I was nine? Grade 4.

These obsessions were my constant companions through those growing-up years. I worried and compared, I dieted and relapsed. I took off a few pounds here, put them back on there. I felt stiff and awkward. In adolescence, I began to wear the shorter skirts and more form-fitting tops my friends were wearing, all the while hoping that people weren't twittering behind my back at how silly the fat girl looked trying to dress like everyone else. In comparison to my slimmer, prettier friends, I believed I was always being judged as wanting. Religion began to play a bigger part in my life but seemed to have nothing to say to my struggles with food and body image. If anything, I imagined that God would also be happier with me if I were skinnier. As I began to contemplate possible leadership in the church, I was sure that the message I would offer would be a lot more compelling to a nonreligious world if I were thin.

My life, beneath the boyfriends, friendship dramas, stress over getting good grades, and negotiations with my parents, was governed by three relentless thoughts:

1. What can I eat next?
2. I just need to lose X number of pounds.
3. Do I look fat?

Having My Cake and Eating It Too

I thought I had discovered the key to the universe when I figured out how to make myself throw up. There was a vision that was just beyond my grasp—a carrot leading me on. It was me in a slinky backless top, my smooth, toned, thin body modestly covered, except that one suggestive area. Along with the image, I could hear the surprised, admiring, even envious comments, "Wow, you look great!" "You've lost weight!" and "How did you do it?"

The idea was first presented to me by a friend when we were first-year university music students. I had eaten too much Mexican food and was feeling sick and bloated as a result.

"Just make yourself throw up," she suggested nonchalantly. Her words were revelatory. I could screw up and there was a way to wipe the slate clean! Back in my dorm later that night, I waited until there was nobody else in the communal washroom and went into one of the stalls. I tried to purge, but as disgusting and bloated as I felt, I couldn't get my gag reflex to work. I went to bed, as I had so many times before, feeling heavy and ashamed.

In the years that followed, the unsuccessful diets kept piling up. Whenever I would make a resolution to restrict my eating, my cravings would correspondingly swell out of control. Out loud, I would blame my dieting failures on genetics. *It's because I am a Smith. Smiths LOVE food.* Inside, however, the more that dieting failed, the more I became convinced that dieting success is what I needed more than anything. I was increasingly desperate to be free of that nine-year-old girl holding in the embarrassment of her overly large stomach.

In my fourth year of university, that whispered suggestion rocketed back to me in a moment of searing insight. I was enjoying a night of board games and overeating with my closest friends. I surveyed the room. There was the friend who seemed able to indulge without gaining weight, and another who had recently lost twenty pounds. "Oh, it was easy," she said when we asked her the key to her success. "I just started walking and I guess the weight came off." Then there were the rest of us who still obsessed about the extra pounds we believed we had to lose. We were implicated by the easy slimness of the other two—clearly, the rest of us had deficits in willpower and self-care. Suddenly I knew the secret. Each of these effortlessly svelte friends would later stick a finger down her throat to get rid of the excess. It was a smart and easy way of having your cake . . . and eating it too.

The first time that I managed to bring back up the bad food I had eaten, I felt that soaring hope that I had felt so many times before. This time would be different. *I was finally going to lose weight.* Bulimia was the ideal boyfriend I had failed to notice until now—the quiet dreamboat who had been standing on the sidelines all along, beckoning me to address my wildest dream and my deepest insecurity by giving up the battle against my favorite security blanket. How had I so long failed to give myself over to this perfect companion?

My body reacted physically to the thrill of this new secret, to the loneliness I was trying to feed, to the addiction I thought I could control by setting it loose. I started overindulging more regularly because I could. I became hungry because the world of food had become available to me, consequence-free. I got hungrier—a deep pit-of-the-stomach, rumbling, obsessive hunger. I woke up thinking about food. I went to bed thinking about food. I would plan out what I was going to eat the next day, and then I would reach the end of a long day of eating unable to face the fact that there was nothing more to stuff into myself. One night, while visiting my grandmother, I wolfed down a four-scoop ice cream sundae topped with two kinds of syrup, chocolate chips, and M&Ms. All I wanted was to feel full. I came to the end of it far too quickly and had to choke back the illogical tears of a spoiled child. The rest of the night stretched endlessly in front of me. There was nothing left to eat until breakfast the next morning.

My hunger was stronger than my gag reflex. I never lost weight. I never got my shining moment in the backless top surrounded by admiring friends asking me how I had managed to drop poundage. I never got to say, "*Oh, it was easy . . .*"

I stopped short of pursuing the extremes of the disease. Laxatives were appealing, for example, as a way to ensure effective purging, but the idea of anyone finding out what I was doing—the possibility of being called out to "get help"—reigned me in. I didn't want to be sick and damaged. I just wanted to eat a bag of Doritos and not have to live with the consequences.

I wasn't losing weight, but for a while there were other compensations. It was a religious experience, one that quickly became the focal point of my day. Originally my plan had been to use purging as an occasional corrective to a mistake, but "binge and purge" instead became something I did regularly behind closed doors. I planned out my mistakes, and I did so knowing that afterward I would be shiny and new again. I would be in lectures, or at choir practice, or out with friends, and I would be thinking about what awaited me later: too many slices of pizza, a bag of chips at the computer, a nauseating number of gummies while studying, all the while knowing that both indulgence and absolution were mine for the taking.

Indulgence and absolution ultimately weren't enough. Weight loss was still the dangling carrot. The harder I tried, the further that carrot seemed to get from me. I became more and more convinced that if I were twenty pounds lighter, if I could just look good wearing one of those backless tops, I would meet my soul mate. I would be recognized and admired. I would be successful and loved. My failure to win the battle over those twenty pounds was a failure of my entire being.

I went to bed every night a mess of conflicting disappointments. I was disappointed to not be thinner. I was disappointed to be hungry. I was disappointed with what I ate that day. I was not exactly disappointed about being somebody who made myself throw up, but I was disappointed it wasn't working better. I was disappointed in myself for not being more committed. The food I had consumed, the emptiness that still ached inside, the acidic burning in my throat from purging, and the obsession about the next day's food choices combined to tie a rock-hard knot of anxiety that weighed down and bloated out every cell of my body.

I did eventually stop. I can guess now that I would have continued much longer down this road, with more damage to my body, if bulimia had yielded what I wanted. But I was about to begin a new chapter of my life. I was graduating with a music degree and beginning seminary in the fall. I had been claimed by a call to priestly ministry when I was fifteen, but had been mostly happy to park my faith life in a tidy and private compartment during college. It was a time for a new beginning. As a smoker might describe their cigarette breaks, binging and purging had become the focus and structure of my day. It wasn't serving me well, but it was nonetheless a supreme act of willpower, enabled by a change of cities, social circles, and studies, to give it up. I felt great reluctance, and I suffered several relapses. By the time I moved to Toronto that fall, I had succeeded in one thing. I had stopped forcing myself to purge.

It felt like the opposite of success. The outward sign of my eating disorder was gone. Inside I was left with one more feeling of failure. The obsessions raged on, but without a physical release. Inside, the life-long pattern of body dis-ease tightened its iron grip.

At War with Our Bodies

Our Eating Disorder

I could tell you about sadness in my life, and I could then blame that sadness for pulling the trigger of bulimia for me—two beloved grandparents dying in the space of a year, the ending of a long-term relationship, the seeming loss of my circle of closest friends as they launched into their own long-term relationships. I could scratch further into the patterns that connected me to my nine-year-old self struggling to be seen and accepted, and my feeling trapped in the emotions and imaginings that put me out of step with most of my classmates, even as I refused to change in order to fit in.

But the more interesting truth about both that time in my life, as well as my childhood, is the happiness. When I now visit London, Ontario, I am flooded with memories of university heartbreak and friendship; hilarious parties and revelatory classes; long, rambling conversations; dalliances and laughter, all set against the backdrop of the discovery and excess a university campus has to offer. The overwhelming intensity of those memories has been worn smooth by the perspective of time into a warm and glowing happiness. Likewise, while I can reflect back on the insecurities of growing up, I will conclude with gladness that my childhood was a safe and nurtured one, teeming with play and shelter and love.

I was happy. That is true. And it is also true that any experience, however minor, of sadness, inadequacy, and embarrassment was written in broken lines and jagged edges across my relationship with my body. I made visible in my body any mental or spiritual dis-ease I experienced. Although I spent many years feeling isolated in that disorder, I now understand that the body is the arena where many of us live out our disorders. There is a visceral, instinctual connection between our stomachs and our emotions. I understand, too, that I was trapped by a seductive belief system designed to ensnare me. I was coddled and encouraged in all of my disordered eating by a whole system of disorder around me.

Tortured by Our Bodies: We Are at War

> The obese body is an expression of excess, decadence, and weakness. . . . It is a losing battleground in a war between willpower and food and metabolism in which you are the ultimate loser. Rarely does a day go by, particularly in the United States, without some new article discussing the obesity epidemic, the crisis. . . . No one wants to be infected by obesity, largely because people know how they see and treat and think about fat people and don't want such a fate to befall them.
>
> —Roxanne Gay, *Hunger*[1]

We have all heard the alarm over the rising rates of obesity and the slew of health problems that accompany extra weight. We are also aware of the perils of the wide variety of fatty, sugary junk food relentlessly marketed to us. Considerable research has been done examining why we overeat, what is causing us to get fat, what foods we should be eating, and which ones we should be avoiding. Countless solutions have been marketed to us, whether in the form of celebrity diets or through government-sponsored health organizations. But across the food industry—junk food, fast food, and diet food—what do our food messages share in common? And what do those messages reveal about our attitudes and beliefs about our bodies and our relationship with food? How do these attitudes feed off one another to keep the food industry booming and us trapped?

I tried a little experiment. I walked into a grocery store one summer Saturday and snapped a picture of every caption about weight loss

---

1. Roxanne Gay, *Hunger: A Memoir of (My) Body* (New York: HarperCollins Publishers, 2017), 122–23.

or celebrity bodies featured on every magazine displayed at the check-out. I limited myself to noting the captions that I could easily see. As I waited to pay for my groceries, here is a cross section of what I found staring me in the face:

- TORTURED BY HER BODY: She's lost 30 lbs in 2 months, but Kim won't leave her house until she gets her bikini body back.
- Jessica: MORE WEIGHT STRUGGLES
- KIM WANTS EVERYONE TO MEET HER BABY! <u>PLUS: HER HOT NEW BODY!</u> (Underline mine)
- Trisha Yearwood: "I'm 35 lbs lighter." Her simple eating plan
- Metabolism—Foods that spark weight loss
- Have a slow metabolism? Your drinking water could be to blame!
- Suddenly Slim—Fall looks that make you look a size smaller
- Lose 23 lbs in 2 weeks—Stubborn fat breakthrough. New research: Even small insulin upticks can prevent weight loss
- Diets That Work: How Jenna lost 23 lbs in 6 weeks
- Love lbs Wow! Eva's new curves
- Mega-Metabolism Smoothie! Fat melting recipe!
- High Fiber = A Slimmer You! Lose 10 lbs in 5 days eating slender-izing "miracle carbs"!
- Weight Loss Secrets No One Ever Tells You

"Tortured by Her Body!"—that first caption from my supermar-ket foray detailed the weight loss struggles of the (complicit? willing? actively participating?) victim Kim Kardashian, and encapsulated a conflict that is on relentless repeat: we are at war with our bodies. Var-ious other celebrities were trotted out to similarly represent the battle-ground. Eva Longoria was one of the week's losers and therefore was mildly taunted for having "love curves," whereas Trisha Yearwood was awarded the medal of honor for losing weight and having a diet to share as well.

We are encouraged to be scandalized by famous people who have put on a few pounds and been foolish enough to be photographed with cellulite. Likewise, we are to be motivated by both the celebrities and the "Average Joes" who have lost extreme amounts of body fat, and to fall for each front-page promise of quick and easy weight loss that will temporarily give us victory over The Bulge.

Had I opened up any of those magazines, I would have found a continuation of the battleground messages, shot at me from other vantage points. The fast-food industry sells quick solutions to the inconvenience of having to feed our bodies. The junk food industry is ready to reward us with tantalizing layers of salt, sugar, and fat for every stress we endure and every celebration we honor. The diet food industry sells long, unpronounceable lists of preservatives and chemicals, along with reductionist promises of how many calories are contained in each offering. Whereas fast and junk foods need strange ingredients to make low-quality products taste irresistible and last on the shelf, diet foods need to manipulate low-calorie, low-fat products into tasting like "the real thing." We are seductively, painstakingly, and thoroughly sold into this war with our bodies, and we are sold it from all sides by industries that have ganged up on us. We buy their weapons willingly, and we wield them against ourselves. We keep relying on the Fast and falling for the Junk, which makes us seek the Diet. The Junk and the Fast and the Diet all reinforce the same battleground messages, and they have physical implications. They also have spiritual implications:

> Our bodies are not to be trusted or listened to, but rather *fooled*.
>
> Our bodies are falling short of the standard set for them; they torture us.
>
> Our bodies threaten us with disappointment and disorder.

We are at war with our bodies.

I Can Win—Salvation for Me

Writer and activist Bill McKibben engaged in his own experiment. In the 1990s, he recorded every available channel on television for twenty-four hours and then watched the 2,184 hours of content. He compared the twenty-four hours of television to spending twenty-four hours in the wilderness. Despite the supposedly wide variety of programming, he had no trouble boiling down the television messages into one primary belief: *You are the center of the universe.*

We may think we live in a secular society, but in fact, what we see in McKibben's research is a relentless religious promise: *I* am saved by getting what *I* need, want, desire, deserve. *Gotta have it*: the essential message of the multi-trillion-dollar advertising industry.

The magazine captions in my experiment give a consistent message of what I need to do to save myself: *A slimmer YOU. Weight loss secrets for YOU. How YOU can dress to look thinner.* But these messages become more effective when they are teamed up with the right partner. At the same time that I am scheming about my strategy for my perfect body, I learn to consume other individuals as nothing more than products—Kim, Trisha, Eva, Jenna are splashed across the front of these magazines for my consumption. I may be the center of the universe, but the body I am seeking is held up to the world for judgment, turned into a product to be labelled "good enough," or, more likely, "needs work." I am taught to obsess about something that I am also taught is fundamentally inadequate.

Secret Knowledge Is Available to Win the War on Our Bodies

We all like a secret. Although the media sell us mass messages, they have an effective knack for intimacy: "Weight loss secrets no one ever tells you"—a chatty celeb like Trisha Yearwood dishes the dirt on her own dieting. They offer promises of exclusivity, even if the promises are mostly illusory. To the list of promises in my sample of magazines, I could add a much longer list of "secret" weight-loss solutions I have tried or that have been shared around the office water cooler, at supper with friends, or across the walls of Facebook. Each has been marketed as the one great key, and each has failed to produce any lasting change in any body I have ever known.

> If you cut out carbs . . . If you separate carbs and proteins . . . If you eat these vitamins . . . If you eat these vitamins in combination with cutting out carbs . . . If you spend twenty minutes a day

on these stretches . . . If you eat flax seed three times a day . . . If you mix in this protein powder . . . If you replace two meals with these milkshakes . . . If you count your calories . . . If you don't eat after 7 p.m. . . . If you eat small amounts regularly . . . If you don't snack . . . If you measure your portions . . . If you buy these portion-controlled meals . . . If you take this pill . . . If you research your blood type . . . If you drink caffeine . . . If you don't drink caffeine . . . If you cut out red meat . . . If you add in low-fat dairy . . . If you cut out dairy . . . If you buy sugar substitutes . . . If you eat honey . . . If you avoid sweets . . . If you drink diet pop . . . If you eat whole grains . . . If you go gluten-free . . .

Gluten free is enjoying its moment in the sun as I write. With it comes both debate and backlash: articles, panel discussions, and television features examine both the science and the experience of gluten-free eating. I grew up when we all feared cholesterol, that mysterious force that we suddenly became aware was part of our food and that could be measured in our bodies, that just as suddenly created a market for "cholesterol free"—a vague, but compelling promise. We believed that things like bacon fat were the demons of the food world, clogging our arteries, giving us heart attacks, killing us off with the ignorance of having not yet discovered nonstick cooking sprays and scientifically manipulated potato chips. Depending on which "expert" you read now, you might discover that returning to the bacon fat is the way to go.

Gluten is the new cholesterol—the supposed key to explaining and solving our fat problems. YouTube boasts a very funny "Pedestrian Question" from *Jimmy Kimmel Live* that sends a camera crew to a popular exercise club in Los Angeles to ask people who don't eat gluten if they know what gluten is. As Kimmel summarizes, gluten is "the thing that we don't eat because someone in our yoga class told us not to."[2]

Once again, we pounce on the "good news." A doctor or movie star has discovered the magic solution, and if I religiously treat my food intake as a carefully ordered formula, if I consume the right

---

2. "Pedestrian Question: What Is Gluten?" *Jimmy Kimmel Live*, May 6, 2014.

combination of products at the right time in the right way, my body will be brought under control.

The fast food, junk food, diet food, health food, and celebrity industries work in concert to keep us dissatisfied with our bodies and subservient to their products. "You are not good enough" combines with "you deserve it" to cycle us between giving in to temptation and feeling badly for doing so. We are ripe for being sold the solution—I only need discipline, the right magic information, and a willingness to part with some of my money to get it and I will unlock the prison door that has trapped me in fat and disease, liberating the thin, vibrant, energetic, invincible body that has been there for me all along.

Is This Just about Girls?

"I have no idea how to eat," a friend confessed to me when I began writing this book. "I might go a whole day without eating, then I binge on the wrong things. I feel guilty. I've been around every dieting block. My whole life I realize I have never known how to just enjoy and be healthy. I have never known how to eat." These words are from a well-educated woman who has the ability to keep up on the available research on healthy eating. She can shop for fresh ingredients and she can cook. She is not mindlessly sucking down bottles of sugary iced tea because she's mistakenly under the impression that if it isn't called "pop" then it must be healthy. She is fit and beautiful, athletic and well dressed.

I have known a lot of beautiful girls, and now women, who openly trash-talk their bodies and speak publicly of all of the flaws that they see in their hips and bellies, thighs and skin. Many of them admit to being lost, frustrated, and despairing in trying to navigate food and diets—except when they happen to be new converts of a diet and are evangelizing others to their discovery. They should be thriving in the blessing of their strong and healthy bodies, but are instead fearful of every bite of food, embarrassed by their inability to get "swimsuit ready," and feel "just five pounds away from my ideal weight." Or, as another friend so disturbingly put it, "Just one stomach flu away." Yikes.

I also know young women who, according to medical standards, need to lose weight. They are already on the verge of suffering joint pain, mobility issues, or diet-induced diabetes. They supposedly have all of the resources and know-how to make much-needed changes, but for a variety of reasons can't make those resources serve the goal of weight loss. Some will admit that food and fat have become a reaction to experiences in which their bodies have been hurt. Others have learned that even the most faithfully followed diets don't necessarily lead to lasting weight loss results. They are oftentimes dismissed: *If she doesn't want to be fat, why doesn't she just* work *at it?* Such words of judgment are dropped from the lips of men and women whose weight is relatively healthy and who want no part in understanding how another's could spiral out of control.

My own confusion in the daily activity of eating is a disturbingly common phenomenon. My longing for illness to force me into weight loss and my desperate discomfort in my body are dynamics that resonate widely. Whether our excess pounds are real or imagined, concern around body weight occupies prime real estate in all too many mental landscapes.

But is it just girls? Girls who haven't yet found a partner? Girls Gen X and younger? We are the ones who were raised within a mass media universe that is relentless in its dieting advice and its campaign of unrealistic expectations for the female body. The media, hocking their multitude of beauty products and "health" solutions, are arguably preying on the vanity of young girls. Cultural analyst and feminist writer Naomi Wolf argues that "The Beauty Myth" is, in fact, intentionally created in order to subjugate the otherwise empowered female to an unattainable standard of beauty. She notes that while women have become more powerful and more liberated, "eating disorders rose exponentially and cosmetic surgery became the fastest-growing specialty . . . and thirty-three thousand American women told researchers that they would rather lose ten to fifteen pounds than achieve any other goal. . . . More women have more money and power and scope and legal recognition than we have ever had before; but in terms of how we feel about ourselves physically, we may actually be worse off than our unliberated grandmothers."

The problem with this analysis is that "eating disorder" becomes equated with the female segment of the population, and we believe that a woman's (young or otherwise) struggle with food is a quest to be beautiful. Instead, statistics suggest a different story. The National Eating Disorder Association in the United States estimates that thirty million people in the U.S. will suffer from an eating disorder at some point in their life. Experts suggest that as many as 30 percent of eating disorder cases are male, but these numbers are consistently underrepresented in official statistics because eating disorders are stereotyped as a "girls' disease."[3] And eating disorders are now listed as having the highest death rate of any psychological illness.[4]

It is more than a question of vanity; it is deadly psychological pain made visible in a vanishing body. Although it makes me livid when "girls' problems" are dismissed because they only affect half of the population—and the half of the population that has traditionally held less power—this isn't just a female issue.

An Even Bigger Problem

Even the seriousness and prevalence of diagnosed eating disorders in our society, however, can be misleading. Anxiety around food is far more pervasive than even these alarming statistics suggest. See if these anecdotes resonate with your experience:

- When I was nine years old and announced I was going on a diet, there was not an adult in my life who suggested it was unnecessary or inappropriate. That might make you assume I was an overweight kid. I wasn't.[5]

- Many of my friends, who were similarly healthy and beautiful and normal, were encouraged, or even forced, to diet by their parents. "I just didn't want you to have the same weight struggles I did," these parents say now. They thought they were doing the right

---

3. Lois Metzger, "What I've Learned about Eating Disorders and Teenage Boys," *The Huffington Post*, June 9, 2013.

4. Ibid.

5. National Eating Disorder Association (NEDA) notes that "40–60% of elementary school girls (ages 6–12) are concerned about their weight or about becoming too fat. This concern endures through life (L. Smolak, "Body Image Development in Childhood," in *Body Image: A Handbook of Science, Practice, and Prevention*, 2nd ed., ed. T. Cash and L. Smolak [New York: Guilford, 2011], *https://www.nationaleatingdisorders.org/sites/default/files/ResourceHandouts/General Statistics.pdf*).

thing, and yet, some of these friends are still suffering the consequences of having starved themselves throughout their teen years with nothing but admiration from their parents for the results their discipline produced.

- Magazines from *Seventeen* for teenaged girls, to *Cosmopolitan* and *Chatelaine* marketed to grown women, to *Zoomer* for the retired generation of women and men, all obsess about food and bodies, whether in offering new diets and workouts, in advertising junk food, or in admiring the bodies of those who are assessed as fit, trim, and therefore beautiful.

- A week never goes by in listening to my favorite public radio station, whose audience is made up of predominantly well-educated and older men and women, without some feature on changing our eating habits, or panels on proper nutrition, obesity and sugar consumption, dieting, vitamin supplements, or weight loss techniques. The segments are featured on talk shows, arts and culture programs, phone-ins, and news updates.

- The men in my life diet. No amount of knowledge of, or commitment to, healthy eating has been able to permanently stave off the demon of extra pounds. Whether male or female, the same pendulum consistently swings between unsustainable restraint and the caving-in to guilt-laden indulgence.

Though the media obsession with perfect bodies fuels the body image problems of many girls and younger women, I am talking about more than the younger demographic, more than a "girls' disease," and definitely more than vanity. When it comes to our relationship with food, the generation gap is remarkably nonexistent. Across the spectrum of male and female, across the lines of the Depression, Boomer, Gen X, Y, Millennial, and Z generations, we see the acceptance of nonstop dieting and a pervasive dissatisfaction with the bodies we have, which has spiraled into three things:

1. An obsessive health consciousness.
2. A shocking and dangerous rise in obesity.
3. A profound sense of alienation and unhappiness in our bodies.

Does It Matter?

Maybe we haven't found the perfect solution to permanent weight loss. Maybe a small percentage of people are making a large amount of money on selling us anxiety and a set of solutions to that anxiety that doesn't particularly work—yet, anyway. Dieting can be approached with the same hopefulness as buying lottery tickets: the big win is always just around the corner.

So what? Maybe there is nothing wrong with obsessing about having the most beautiful body I possibly can. Maybe we only think there is something indecent about wanting great figures because of long-held prudishness around sex and skin. Maybe we live in a time of supreme liberation from fat and cravings and vitamin deficiencies, and maybe the right diet is paving the way . . .

. . . Except that there are far-reaching ramifications to embracing these messages. What we see in magazine headlines, television programming, and fad diets looks like celebrity news, mindless entertainment, and nutritional advice. In fact, these various media all work together to deliver the consistent spiritual message that our bodies are untrustworthy, and to be saved we need the right diet and a smaller waistline. If we are to reclaim joy and health in our bodies, then, we need a different spiritual message—and we need it because this war on bodies is making us *all* sick.

You Are *Not* the Center of the Universe: The Wider Consequences

It is not just that I am relentlessly taught to both obsess over and distrust my body. I am also given the subtle and consistent message that bod*ies* do not matter—third-world bodies, animal bodies, the complex multibody chain of life. Although our actions suggest that our individual bodies are inconvenient garbage dumps with which we are at war, the food industry also promises that nothing trumps the body's individual desire, individual convenience, individual lifestyle, when deciding food choices. *You are the center of the universe* isn't just the message we get from television; it's the message we take into our very flesh in what and how we eat.

We seek our convenient food and stuff our landfills with appalling amounts of plastic packaging. We obsess about lean proteins and low-carb diets. We crave fast, generic meat, cleverly prepared to disguise any resemblance to an actual animal. And our demand is both created and met by massive industrial farms and slaughterhouses, raising animals in appalling conditions, pumping them full of hormones and cheap feed to maximize profits and yield. We import our food products from the developing world in mass quantities, throwing out a staggering 40 percent of our available food in North America, while people living in other parts of the world starve. Meanwhile, the collateral carbon dioxide damage of food transportation costs chokes our airways and waterways.

Our attitude to the individual body and our attitude to our collective body are fundamentally linked. When we name our own bodies as inadequate or disappointing, we also create a culture of disrespect for the bodies within which we exist and have life. As the wants of an individual body justify harming the systems of life within which it exists, the loop is completed—we further disrespect the individual body, the individual body which actually does not and cannot live in isolation.

Which brings it all back to Me: Me at the center of the universe. This is the key component of this destructive individualism. It is not just that my body is worthless, untrustworthy, and a failure. It is also that our communal bodies are treated the same. Care for both self and world is seriously compromised when we are unencumbered by any responsibility to anything or anyone other than ourselves.

If . . .

If you have experienced our society's obsession with perfect bodies as something less than liberating; if you have tried the various paths of dieting and found yourself locked in an unwinnable war; if you have experienced a frustrating search down a dead-end path in the food we eat and the way we eat it; if you have had a glimpse, here and there, now and then, of how your body might be flawed and imperfect and beautiful and powerful, then maybe you want to explore a different possibility.

If you feel drawn to be something other than an isolated, alien-ated individual; if you suspect that somehow, somewhere along the line, we have to figure out how our lives are not just for ourselves; if you have looked thoughtfully at the world around you and won-dered at the destruction we are wreaking, the empty void that we keep expanding as we increasingly serve only the individual; then yes, challenging the status quo about our relationship with food and bodies does matter.

Our problem with our bodies does not boil down to too many calories. There are certainly physical problems gripping us, like obesity and eating disorders, but these physical problems are fundamentally linked to imbalance and untruth in the mind and heart. In the spirit.

Although the most powerful and pervasive messages by which we live are now delivered from the realm of the secular, it is from a realm that is often now regarded as "fringe" where we find a different choice.

The Christian Alternative: The Scandal of the Incarnation

"The Word became flesh and lived among us," the Gospel of John preposterously claims in its opening poetic description of Jesus. It is an explicit statement of a current of controversy running throughout the four gospel accounts of Jesus's life. It is the belief, finally and wildly embraced by early Christians, that was (and still is) so scandalous, not only to those not following Jesus, but sometimes even to those who are. Whereas "chili con carne" means "chili with meat," Incarnation means "*God* with meat." We believe that we discover who God is through the bodily, fleshly, meaty person of Jesus.

God was revealed to us in the body. In Jesus, our physical existence is forever marked as good, as valued, as holy, as bearing the possibil-ity of revealing truth and life, as intimately connected to the world—the definition of bodily existence is relationship. It is a scandalous and messy proposition. The Christian Church has at times pushed back against its own teaching, finding ways of presenting instead a neatly packaged disregard for our own physical existence—the baser physical existence must be brought under heel by the elevated life of spirit.

And yet, when we actually look to Jesus, we find a man, a teacher, a witness, a Way who tells us that our bodies can lead us to God. God's promise was delivered to the people of Israel by the prophet Jeremiah, "I will put my law within them, and I will write it on their hearts" (Jer. 31:33). Jesus took Jeremiah's promise one step further: the love of God is written *in our bodies*. More specifically, Jesus located this spiritual path and spiritual knowledge not just in our bodies, but in our stomachs—how and what we eat, the hunger inside us. He broke this basic act of survival open for his followers and showed the way of relationship, community, healing, and union. Right relationship with hunger and body was the marker for right relationship with God. Bread, water, wine, banquet, hunger, thirst, breaking, and sharing became the signposts for the kingdom of God.

Jesus did not "come among us" to reform a diet industry. But his life and death and re-creation offer an understanding of bodily life that speaks far outside the constraints of the culture and time in which Jesus lived and acted. More than that, in coming to know Jesus, we begin to realize that the destruction and false promises of what this life is for, as proclaimed in our unhealthy relationship with food, simply cannot go unaddressed. In the wake of how Jesus speaks to us here and now, he offers another possibility—a life-giving, truthful, time-tested possibility for how we can be in relationship with our bodies, with the physical world around us and with God. That possibility starts with and is revealed in food.

Holding His Feet

Some things improved when I began my first year of seminary. I met my future husband, Dan. It is not that I needed Prince Charming in order to achieve some mythical happily ever after. I will unabashedly say, however, that life became better when I had somebody to really talk to, when I was finally able to have those conversations that had been burning inside of me for what seemed like all of my life.

I stopped watching TV. We didn't have a television on our floor of the residence and there was never enough time to seek one out somewhere else in the building. Being forced to "tune out" helped too.

Although when I started training to be a priest I was led by little more than a vague sense that it felt right—even when I was mostly uncertain of what I believed or where I saw my life going—I quickly settled into the most exhilarating studies I had ever encountered. My life had been a set of jagged puzzle pieces. Nothing about who I was or where I was going seemed to naturally fit together. Suddenly, a few of those pieces turned out to fit together perfectly.

Loneliness and isolation had been significant companions of my eating disorder and my disorder "fed" them, amplifying rather than alleviating their presence. When I started seminary, I had given up throwing up. With regret. I had found much comfort in both the bad choices and the regular ability to physically purge myself of those choices. Still, it was good to start in a new place, with new people, with new direction, and leave behind that secret. I no longer had the outward signs of an eating disorder.

But the obsessions never left me alone; they were as familiar to me as my own family members. It wasn't so much that I didn't know how to rid myself of them, rather it was that it didn't occur to me that there was a possibility of life without them. Every choice I made for sweets or fries, every time the hunger got the better of me and I gave in to cookies or muffins, every weakness I showed on the battlefield of the War for Thinness made me feel the full weight of failure and guilt. My mental pendulum continued to swing, more gently than before perhaps, but still there was a constant movement between the disgust I felt whenever I looked in the mirror seeing only extra weight and the wild hope that *this* time I would find the motivation and discipline to make the diet work and to drop pounds.

This went on for another three years. In the meantime, Dan and I married. In conjunction with that momentous event I also received my other long-hoped-for desire. I lost weight for the wedding and, more importantly, I did it without dieting and worrying. I was too busy with the fear and trembling surrounding this lifelong commitment I was about to make to allow my body-image demons to occupy much mental energy. It was a taste of grace.

It was the comments afterward, the surprised admiration ("Wow, where have you disappeared to?" and "My goodness, you've lost a lot of weight!") that grabbed me and pulled me under that familiar blanket of despair again. It was what I had wanted for so long, yet when I got it, it was devastating. I felt judged in how I had looked before; I was fearful of re-gaining the weight.

On April 3, 2004, Dan and I came home from a family birthday party. We had enjoyed wings and pizza and various appetizers. Dessert was an enormous carrot cake with cream cheese icing. We each had a generous slice at the party, and we gladly brought home two big pieces to enjoy later. It was exactly the way I liked carrot cake—no raisins, loaded with nuts, and topped with thick cream cheese icing. We ate the extra pieces before bed.

"Did you see that little girl at the party?" I remarked to Dan as we brushed our teeth and prepared for sleep. "I don't understand why her parents would let her keep loading up her plate with all of that greasy food. She is going to have problems later in life if they're not careful." As is usually the case when we snark about others, it did little to alleviate the disgust I felt with myself.

In our new life, I loved that Dan and I assumed time for prayer at the beginning and ending of the day and had set up a small prayer area in our bedroom. I settled myself into one of the two chairs and pulled out the small brown leather prayer book that guided me through the daily lectionary, which is a two-year cycle of readings appointing portions of scripture for Christians to read every day of the year. Because it takes the choice of scripture out of the individual's hands, it is remarkable how deftly that random element of readings chosen long ago by someone else allows the working of the Spirit to speak into our lives. At the suggestion of my spiritual director, Audrey, I was experimenting with a new form of visualization prayer.

The reading for that night was of Jesus's encounter with the blind man, Bartimaeus (Mark 10:46–52). Bartimaeus, though blind, had a piercing ability to see Jesus for who he was. Jesus could save him, and he hollered unashamedly from the roadside: "Son of David, have mercy on me!" He was told to hush up. Nobody thought that his matter was worthy of Jesus's attention. Jesus was predictably stubborn in the face of his disciples' deeply entrenched need to herd him into the pen of respectability and to shield him from the indecent. He called the man over. Bartimaeus couldn't run to him fast enough. Jesus asked the pointed question, "What do you desire?" "My rabbi, I want to see," Bartimaeus said without hesitation, all guards down. Jesus pronounced him healed and Bartimaeus continued on his journey.

I got into bed and closed my eyes to picture myself in the story. The details began to fill in for me. I knew that Jesus had better things to do than notice me, but I shouted out my simple plea for mercy anyway. The news that the Master is calling me over comes as a lightning shock that sends me running to this man, whose face I can't bear to even imagine. When those words are spoken to me—"What do you desire?"—I find myself facedown on the ground, desperately holding Jesus's feet, unable to look up. I am opened by the weight of a great love I have never so fully known. I don't say anything. I know what I want, and I know Jesus understands. I want to be healed.

I fell asleep holding his feet.

I woke up with a desperate, body shuddering, sweat-and-tears kind of nausea and ran to stick my head in the toilet. It was not the controlled demolition of my previous bulimia. My stomach was violently revolting against everything it had been in contact with. I miserably vomited for the next twenty-four hours. Although Dan and I had eaten the same food and shared the same living-breathing space, he neither came down with food poisoning nor stomach flu.

Through my sudden sickness, I had the unshakeable sense that I had been heard, and I had been answered. Something dark and malignant was being physically purged. I had tasted this bile all my life, never believing I had any choice in the sour flavor it adhered to everything I consumed. Now, as it viciously exited my body, I wondered if I might be tasting it for the last time.

Born Hungry

J esus has something to say to my relationship with food, but the more important thing I have discovered is that Jesus has something to say about *our* relationship with food. The one thing is inextricably linked with the other. Salvation is not a merely individual offering.

My problems—obsessing about thinness and sticking my fingers down my throat—are modern-day, first-world problems. They tend to be judged harshly as vain and selfish individual choices. I am reminded of a crass punch line I heard once in a sitcom episode. A character who we were to understand as superficial and self-involved says to her friend, "Order me dessert, I'm going to go throw up."

In the face of our modern-day judgments, Jesus has a vested interest in the relationship within and between individual bodies, from those days along the Galilean lakeshore to today. Jesus knows that food matters, that what we eat and how we eat communicates vital information about the health and well-being of individuals, communities, and our world. I can speak personally to the surprising experience of finding that my little life was brought into the attention and care of the life of God in the flesh, and I can also attest to the fact that any healing I have received has never been just about me. Jesus heals the individual by restoring the individual to their place within relationship and community.

Let's examine that right place where human existence is configured, and then how those fundamental human truths were woven into the sacred story that formed Jesus and informed his teaching.

Emotional Eating

In my favorite secondhand bookstore, I came across a title that I couldn't resist—*Women, Food and God: An Unexpected Path to Almost Everything*. Geneen Roth is the author of what turned out to be a self-help book detailing a way of getting and maintaining a healthy body weight by learning to listen to your body rather than dieting. Although the book promises that thoughtful eating will also lead to spiritual enlightenment, she says very little about what sort of God our food would actually connect us to and why. As is the case with many people, negative past experiences of religion had tainted her perspective. The faith she eventually grew into therefore avoids the particularities of any one religious tradition, and she instead broadly defines God as, "a vast expanse that we cannot penetrate with our minds."[1] Although I have no reason to suspect she isn't sincere, she does end up subscribing to a religious understanding that would be most akin to a restaurant menu—one picks and chooses, from a variety of options, the attributes one wants in a deity, along with the spiritual practices and outcomes one finds most appealing. And while that might be the only path she feels she can embrace, the unfortunate ramification is that it entirely buys into the message we are most used to hearing: *I am the center of the universe; salvation is merely about me.*

That isn't to say that the eating practices she describes aren't valuable. I would even agree with some of them. I note Roth's work because of one of her most seemingly sensible suggestions: only eat when you are hungry. She argues that much of our disordered eating stems from using food as a way to avoid feeling: "Eat what you want when you are hungry and feel what you feel when you're not."[2]

---

1. Geneen Roth, *Women, Food and God: An Unexpected Path to Almost Everything* (New York: Simon & Schuster, 2010), 25.

2. Ibid., 101.

Every women's magazine selling every kind of diet will tell you the same thing. Don't eat emotionally. Don't eat out of boredom, sadness, grief, depression, worry, or stress. What I am about to say might seem strange. I agree with Roth that food can be improperly used as a way of numbing pain, and I know that learning to listen to the body is an important learning on the path to wellness. Yet Roth actually prescribes something that is impossible. It is impossible to not eat emotionally. It is impossible to eat only out of pure physical need.

Yes, we eat to numb pain. Yes, the way that we feed our bodies can be a way of making our inner pain visible. Yes, we easily learn how to transfer emotions onto the food we eat. And yes, this can lead to disorder, obesity, and profound discomfort in our bodies. But why? Why is eating emotional? And why might knowing this core truth—*eating is emotional*—lead us to hope and healing?

Which Brings Us to Jesus—and Us

The gospel—the Good News story of Jesus's life—introduces us to a somewhat nefarious and difficult person: a man who is born a bastard and dies a criminal, who challenges and provokes, and who loves and is loved in between these distasteful bookends. And somehow, those who came to follow him insisted that knowing Jesus allowed them to know God.

We meet Jesus in relationship. We meet Jesus for the sake of community. But God understood "the medium is the message" long before twentieth-century communications philosophy would catch up. If we meet Jesus in relationship and for the sake of community, we also discover that Jesus *himself* is relationship, Jesus *himself* is formed in community—as we are too. Our own stories extend far beyond our individual memory banks into patterns woven into the fabric of our beings.

In order to understand something as complicated and yet as basic as our relationship with food, we need to go back to our own beginnings, to our first stories. It is out of my experience as a mother that I finally understand something of the instincts and possibilities hardwired into each of us. But as we bring our eating habits into dialogue with Jesus, I take us first to *his* beginning, to the stories that formed him and his unique relationship with food.

The Israelites

Jesus didn't invent a connection between God and food. He learned it. Jesus's people—the Jewish people—built their lives on the understanding that their history was tied to God's invitation and action among them. Jesus was formed by this story and proclaimed the Good News from inside of it. It is a history of relationship, and it is a story of human hunger.

Thousands of years before he would be born to a brave peasant girl in a barn, Jesus's people were slaves in Egypt, living under a tyrannical king. They were cogs in the machine of Egyptian industry. They were understood as useful tools to be managed and controlled for the benefit of those who were considered to count.

God sees things differently.

The Jewish people are to forever remember the eve of their liberation. On that first Passover, described so vividly in the book of Exodus, judgment and darkness were descending. It was a night of terrible tragedy for those who insisted they could ignore the humanity of the people on whose backs they had become prosperous. The night was made sacred, and a connection reforged, through a meal of roasted lamb and freshly baked bread.

The people ate. They were scared, uncertain, and on the verge of the unknown. But they ate. They ate for practical reasons. They would need strength for the journey ahead. They ate for spiritual reasons too. They ate to know that God was with them. They ate to bind themselves to God as God was binding each of them to one another. They ate as an act of faith in the face of all the terror that surrounded them. They ate to realize a new possibility, to enact the freedom that, against all odds, God was offering to them. The meal was to be shared in all of its detail as the foundation of this emerging people's unique identity in relationship with God. Yet this meal also signified the more general meanings that human beings have, throughout history, understood meals to carry: reconciliation, community, sacrifice, covenant, trust, and nourishment.

The celebration of the Passover meal would, countless generations later, take center stage as Jesus's life came to its critical conclusion. He sat down with his disciples on the night before his death, and he shared in the meal of his ancestors. It was significant that it took prominence at that juncture because it had formed Jesus's life all along. Every year, Jesus and his family and community made the pilgrimage to Jerusalem to be part of remembering—reliving—that night. We will talk more about the Last Supper in a later chapter.

There is another meal that deeply influences Jesus's ministry and which can serve us in reimagining our own relationship with food. This second meal acts not just as a formational narrative for the Israelites, but also serves as metaphor for our universal human journey.

Manna for Newborns

After the Passover and their escape from Egypt, the people of Israel wandered in the wilderness on their way to the Promised Land. They were no longer slaves, but they had not yet learned what it meant to be free. In the midst of their burning anxiety, with the great weight of the unknown bearing down on them, their focus narrowed on one key concern: they were hungry. They lashed out at Moses, arguing that he had liberated them only so they could die of starvation in the desert.

There is something primal about the wilderness experience of the Israelites. They had been shunted down the birth canal of their liberation into a new identity. They were uncoordinated, overwhelmed, and reacting mostly on the level of instinct. They were like newborns, and they responded to all of the terror and uncertainty like any healthy newborn does: they cried for food. As they cried, they encountered the world around them, their choices in that world, and where those choices would lead them. At its worst, their hunger compelled them to forge a golden calf in a midnight fire when they had come to believe they were alone, and that gods and food could be created and manipulated by people disconnected from anything more meaningful than their single selves. Their choice, they would discover, led to death.

In contrast, there was a second choice that led to life. God offered them a sweet and mysterious heaven-sent food; this manna was God's response to their cries of hunger and fear. It came with the dew of

sunrise, a sweet flakey substance that could be shaped into bread or
cakes. It was provided for them each morning as a blessing. The Israelites were to gather it, taking only as much as they needed for their families for that day. They enjoyed the manna for the first few mornings.
Then they got smart. They began to hoard it. They didn't trust that
God would continue to provide for their needs. They had learned
the lesson we teach still: there is not enough. They were thinking
ahead, planning for the scarcity that was inevitable. But they received
a surprise. Anything they took beyond what they needed turned to
maggot-infested waste. God taught them their new identity by feeding them exactly what they needed, exactly as much as they needed,
and in a way that made it clear that the source of their nourishment
was the One who gave them life in the first place. When they finally
found their way to the Promised Land and began to fashion themselves
more concretely into God's people, God laid before them two options:
live or die.

They could live according to the ways of God and teach the promise and love of God one generation to the next, or they could go the
way of idolatry, settling for less than the living God, and allow their
hunger to lead them to anxiety, each individual only for themselves. It
was not that God would punish them for choosing the second way, but
that the natural consequence of this second way was destruction.

Firstfruits

One of the first acts of settling into this new land was to celebrate the
Passover meal. They instituted the practice of annually retelling the
story of their liberation from slavery in Egypt through the sharing of
lamb and unleavened bread—not just remembering the story, but *participating* in it. Although few of the initial group from the liberation
forty years prior were still present, the story of freedom belonged to
everyone. It continued to be their story from that first Passover through
to Jesus. And even through to us.

God no longer provided for their daily needs through the manna.
They graduated from this baby food to feeding themselves from the
produce of the land. But along with the Passover, they were meant to

remember and participate in the teachings of the manna. As they prepared to till the land and reap the harvests, they were given this dual practice of sacrifice and offering. At every harvest they offered the first-fruits back to God, the first blessings of all God had given them. And as they offered, they were to tell their story:

> A wandering Aramean was my ancestor; he went down into Egypt and lived there as an alien, few in number, and there he became a great nation, mighty and populous. When the Egyptians treated us harshly and afflicted us, by imposing hard labor on us, we cried to the LORD, the God of our ancestors; the LORD heard our voice and saw our affliction, our toil, and our oppression. The LORD brought us out of Egypt with a mighty hand and an outstretched arm, with a terrifying display of power, and with signs and wonders; and he brought us into this place and gave us this land, a land flowing with milk and honey. So now I bring the first of the fruit of the ground that you, O LORD, have given me. (Deut. 26:5–10)

They knew their history to be a humble one. They knew what it felt like to be vulnerable, to be "aliens in a strange land," to be enslaved, to be lost. They knew God had provided for them. In their food they recognized their relationship with God and how they were bound to God's people and God's world through God's generosity.

One piece of manna, we are told, was preserved in the Ark of the Covenant, the Israelites' portable temple, as a symbol of God's faithful presence and love for them. The road ahead was often bumpy. The Hebrew Scriptures detail in epic proportions the struggle of this people to trust in the identity conferred on them in the manna, and in the lamb and bread of Passover: people who were free and loved and fed.

Whenever they found their end of the covenant hard to keep, the prophets issued a stirring reminder, "Stop eating that which does not satisfy and receive the good food of God, without cost!" (Isa. 55:1–2). The people of faith we meet on the pages of scripture are startlingly like us. They have tasted, eaten, and digested their true identity. It is hardwired into their bodies, minds, and spirits. Yet it is still easy to choose junk—to eat it . . . to be it.

Emotional Eating

So far in this chapter I have made two claims: eating is emotional and the Israelites' manna serves as metaphor for the universal human experience. Such claims take clearer shape when grounded in personal experience. Let me share mine. On the one hand, I can look back at my bulimia and see that I was lonely and sad. In the absence of better strategies to work through difficulties, I turned to the comforting embrace of food, the reliable pleasures of tasting and eating, and then erasing.

On the other hand, I wasn't just working through difficult emotions. I was also hungry. When my grandfather died, I was hungry. When the dating world turned out to be almost as bad as a bad relationship, I got hungrier still. The more that I tried to control my hunger, the more it controlled me. The worse that I felt about myself and my bad food choices, the deeper and more real that growl in the pit of my stomach became.

I was thoroughly indoctrinated into that core dieting advice: "Only eat when you are hungry." And yet, knowing that did not allow me any measure of control. It only served to add one more failure on my list of all of the things that felt wrong about my life and for which food offered me comfort.

It was many years later when I would begin to appreciate that emotional eating wasn't a failure on my part. We are born this way.

Hunger and Love

I had just given birth to my daughter Cecilia and was full of new-mother hormones. I was sleep deprived and scared. I had no idea what I was doing, and doing the right thing had never mattered so much. In the overwhelming expanse of all that I suddenly did not know, my anxious mind settled on one worry—*my daughter won't stop eating!* I was breastfeeding, and while I had been prepared for the fact that my newborn was unlikely to adhere to the kind of four-hour eating schedule that had once been touted as the norm, I was increasingly concerned by her insatiable appetite. I called my midwife, already mentally packing my bags to make a rushed trip to the hospital, and I explained the situation.

"She's hungry?" my midwife asked. "That's great!" Then she added, "Feed her."

I muddled my way through those early days. I learned about following my baby's signs, sitting still and being present and nourishing to this new creature in my life. It was only much later that the penny dropped. My child was hungry. The one and only survival instinct with which Cecilia had come equipped had shifted into high gear. She was eating, and therefore she was living. She had been safe, warm, and close in the dark world of my womb. She had been shunted into a bright, open, loud, and unknown reality. She was responding to this terror and uncertainty by crying for food. As I held her and fed her, she invested herself fully into the project of survival, and more than that, of life.

In a 1987 scientific discovery, a group of researchers from the Karolinska Institute observed a phenomenon they named the "breast crawl." A newborn infant, seemingly helpless in every respect—eyesight undeveloped, gross and fine motor skills at a bare minimum, not even strong enough to hold its head up on its neck—will, if left alone, follow a clear and discernible pattern of behavior that will result in that newborn finding their food source—their mother's breast—and initiating feeding. The baby is literally hardwired in those first moments of life to do nothing other than use all five senses, every ounce of strength, to "crawl" toward milk.

The baby continues, in their first days and weeks, to develop the muscle and brain power to respond to the world around them, and as that development happens at its lightning pace, they maintain one constant. They react to every fear, every need, every discomfort, with the desire to feed. From the beginning, that core instinct is inextricably linked to much more than their physical needs. As they feed, they are also held. Their skin touches the skin of another. They initiate eye contact, the gaze of the Loving falling on the beloved. This brand-new life chooses survival, and built into that physical survival are the gifts—the *necessities*—of relationship, touch, and love.

Cecilia's first instinct led her to eat from her mother's body, and as she did this insatiably and relentlessly, we fell in love with each

other. Emotional eating is good, natural, holy. It forms the foundation of human life, which, from the outset, is clearly relational. Relationship and survival cannot be separated from one another; food is
programmed to carry not just nourishment, but deep and powerful
emotional content.

I don't remember my own infant experiences of breastfeeding. And
yet, at the same time, I clearly do. What else was I doing in those dark
obsessive adult days if not trying desperately to connect? I was trying to
crawl my way toward a warm body that would hold me, feed me, and
show me that I was loved. I might remember nothing of that first year
of my life, but the experience I no longer remember shaped me forever.

Thank God

Only eat when you are hungry. Don't eat emotionally. It sounds like
simple and reasonable advice. And it shows a complete forgetfulness
of how human life actually works, what human life is actually for.
Eating *is* emotional. It is emotional from the outset and for good
reason. Emotional eating is built into the agenda of survival. Telling
someone to not eat emotionally makes as much sense as telling someone to breathe less. Breathing and eating are our primary instincts.
Thank God.

Thank God for lungs insisting that their craving for air be continually satisfied. Thank God for nourishing our bodies in a way that
directly expands our capacity for giving and receiving love.

Yet knowing that eating is emotional does not mean we are
trapped. It does not mean my addiction to food and my disordered
eating had to be the last words on my life, or that our futile attempts
at filling our empty souls by stuffing our faces with junk have to be the
last words on our collective lives.

What was it the prophets said? *Why do you keep eating that which
is not food?* Those prophets have continually called the people to
remember the lessons they learned on their wilderness journey, in the
bread rained down from heaven on their newborn cries. Emotional
eating has the capacity to teach us something, to remake us into who
we truly are.

Milk and Manna

I was terrified by the full-body requirement of being a new breast-feeding mother. I knew that having children would change my life. I knew that I was getting into a commitment unlike anything I had ever experienced before. What I didn't know is that it would, for a time, be all-consuming. I thought that I could occasionally steal an evening away with my husband and leave Cecilia in the care of my mother and a few breast-milk bottles. I thought my husband could look after her every now and then and I could take a couple of hours to shop or see a friend. I resisted the truth that those first few months would work most effectively if I could surrender and be present.

More than that though, I was haunted by messages I knew all too well about how we can get locked into bad habits, about how we can get spoiled by having all that we want. Again, I wasn't under the illusion that babies should adhere to some rigid schedule of feeding, but for the first few months of Cecilia's life, she fed constantly—five or ten minutes between feedings from 5 p.m. to 10 p.m. every night. Surely that kind of neediness couldn't go unchallenged. Surely I was teaching my daughter the wrong things by giving in to her demands. I wasn't scared that the next few months were going to seriously restrict my freedom. I was scared that I might be setting up an entire lifelong relationship with a child who has learned that she could ask for everything and expect to receive it.

"There are no bad habits for newborns," my midwife tried to tell me. "There is only survival." We interpret a baby's needs and desires in light of our own adult experience. But of course, their needs are pure in a way that we have mostly forgotten. They want milk. They don't want soy milk, or chocolate milk, or a frozen daiquiri with a little umbrella in it. They don't want a decaf-skim-no-foam-double-espresso-latte. They want milk, and in wanting that milk, they want to be loved and safe. They want to establish a relationship. As they are wanting, they are also becoming their particular identity: beloved.

Jesus's ancestors in faith, the Israelites, were also learning and becoming. They received the manna on demand, as much as they needed and wanted, at no cost. They had to relearn their identity.

They were not slaves; they were free. They were not oppressed; they were nurtured. They were not nobodies; they were beloved somebodies.

As I fed Cecilia, I learned. I learned the mysteries of a proper latch and the healing properties of cabbage leaves. As I listened to my midwife explain the miracles of breast milk, I heard a note of wonder catching in her voice. A newborn that is breastfed cannot be overfed. A mother can meet every demand that her baby has. She can feed them when they are hungry, but she can also feed them when they are scared or in pain or tired or fussy, and the baby's body and mother's milk will adjust so that there is no excess, so that the baby has exactly the right amount of energy and builds exactly the right amount of muscle and fat.

The Israelites of the Hebrew Scriptures likewise were given exactly what they needed at the hand of the One who knew them and their needs better than they did. They were not allowed to take more than they needed, to live in fear that the supply of generosity and care would run out. They had to surrender and trust. Of course, the manna was for a season. Eventually, it had to stop. The people came through the wilderness and were called to establish the Promised Land.

The fear that my life would forever be restricted by the every-ten-minute needs of Cecilia seems like a lifetime ago as I watch her now, going to school, writing songs, enjoying sleepovers at friends' houses, saying and doing things that come from the unique person she is and wants to be, and not from anything I initiated.

Notice my language—neither Cecilia nor the people of Israel become independent. Independence is a modern illusion. Human beings are not independent. Much of the pain and poison in our world is created because individuals believe themselves independent from the world around them. Our lives begin with the instinct for eating. Our lives are sustained by eating. Eating is an act of relationship. It is a constant reminder that we need life from outside of ourselves so that we can have life.

The Christian faith defines *person* as a "relational being." Spiritually and emotionally we rely on the witness of our faith to verify this claim. But physically we need no proof. Physically our lives are very clear: they exist in relationship. Manna and breast milk do not teach independence. They teach relationship. Right relationship. Food grounds newborn life in right relationship.

The particular gift of being human is not just that we can receive love, that we can know ourselves as beloved. The particular gift of being human is that we can receive love in order that we might also learn how to give it. The purpose of the manna in the wilderness, the purpose of demand-feeding a newborn, is not to infantilize people, to lock them into an endless cycle of greed and selfishness, but rather to lay the secure foundation out of which the fullness of humanity can be experienced and expressed.

The Israelites began to shape the new community that they had been called into being. Many of the guidelines found in those early books of the Bible sound confusing and irrelevant to our modern ears. But the underlying theme is that they would be a people who sheltered and cared for the vulnerable because these were people who knew what it was to be vulnerable. Strangers were to be welcomed because "you were aliens in the land of Egypt" (Exod. 22:21). Practices of generosity were to be enacted because their wilderness journey founded them in a story of God's provision, of receiving all that they had at the hands of God.

We hope for a similar kind of direction in our children as we shepherd and feed them through babyhood. We want them to know they are loved, but we do our children no favors if that is where our teaching ends. We also want them to learn to be loving. We want them to feel safe and protected, and ultimately a parent's job involves balancing that protection with freedom, with communicating to them that they have lives built on a foundation of trust, so that they can then be entrusted with their own unfolding responsibilities.

The foundational story of a people coming to know the God of freedom and generosity and growing into their identity as God's children is at the center of our human life. Before memory, before words or understanding, before acquiring any skills, before our neural pathways have begun to form rational thought, we are born hungry.

Emotional Eating and Jesus

From the beginning of our lives, the most important emotional information is communicated to us through the act of eating. From the beginning of Jesus's formational spiritual story, food addressed fear and uncertainty, communicated love and protection, enabled compassion and care, and created community and bound a people to one another and to God.

Noting that eating is emotional, though, does not mean that my eating cardboard-like cookies and excessive amounts of high-fat and high-sugar foods to try and fill myself up emotionally and spiritually should be accepted as a mere reflection of ingrained human instinct. I was trapped. But I would have done well to understand that while my hunger was a natural and appropriate response to the barrage of feelings I was experiencing, there were other ways of addressing this appetite than the destructive ones I chose.

When the Jewish prophets asked, "Why do you eat that which is not bread?" they were identifying an age-old problem. There will always be opportunities to feed ourselves with stuff that does not satisfy. There has always been profit in offering junk to feed people's hunger. We know that today better than we have ever known it. And we are realizing the consequences of having so much of this junk available and attractive for the masses to mindlessly consume, never having to identify or address our real hunger.

Jesus blazed onto the scene of first-century Palestine, and he understood his people's story of hunger. He was formed by the scriptural accounts of the unleavened bread, of the manna raining from heaven. He saw the hunger of his own day, heard his people crying out for food and protection. He knew his own hunger and its capacity to lead to truth, life, God. He recognized idolatry and how hunger could be misused, how it could lead to destruction.

We can read the women's magazines with their unrealistic advice to avoid "emotional eating" and then add guilt to the list of emotions already associated with our eating habits. Or, we can look to Jesus, to the wisdom and practices he offers, to how following him can unlock our understanding of hunger and love, to how our hunger and love can be put into the service of life.

chapter

5

Feeding the Emptiness

There was a push toward "anorexia awareness" when I was growing up. I read more than one teen novel that delved into the
disease, describing in vivid detail a young woman who had
stopped eating, her hip bones jutting painfully out of her increasingly
hollowed-out body, though she inexplicably saw only fat and failure in
the mirror.

The pages of *Seventeen* and *YM*—the particularly destructive magazine options presented to my generation of young women, full of
so-called empowering messages while focusing obsessively on consuming
the right products and attracting cute boys—were quick to jump on the
band wagon. They featured stories told from the viewpoint of teenage
girls recovering from the illness, recounting what led them down that
path, exploring what it meant, and offering contact information for available help. Other articles, not dealing specifically with eating disorders,
encouraged us to feel good about our bodies, to understand that we came
in unique sizes and shapes, that we were not all built like supermod-
els. And then the glossy, colorful, enticing pages that followed resound-
ingly told us, "*This is a lie.*" Only one size sells the seductive promises of
beauty and sex appeal that fund magazines: Size Thin.

In the beginning of my teen years (the early 1990s), the message I
got was that size 6 was perfect. Midway through the decade, size 0 was
the new ideal. We pushed back: "How is this even attractive?" "Who
wants to look like a preadolescent boy?" "I *like* having curves!" But the

39

tsunami of images defining the parameters of beauty claimed the upper hand in our collective psyche.

In a radio interview, best-selling novelist Lionel Shriver reached the conclusion that "we all have eating disorders." When questioned on her seemingly vague and controversial claim, she elaborated, "I'm upset by how much time—and this is no longer just a female problem—people are spending anguishing about food. Either planning what to eat or regretting what you did eat. I'm upset by the sheer waste of energy of what is, of course, about physical appearance."[1]

There is a lot of anguish around food. And yet, Shriver is wrong in concluding that it is only an issue of physical appearance. Physical appearance is merely where our deeper anxieties most naturally find a place to make themselves at home.

I remember one article about a girl recovering from anorexia. Her treatment involved seeing a therapist who asked her to name all of the responsibilities she believed she carried. For every responsibility, the therapist threw a pillow at her. She soon found herself standing in a sea of pillows. Her life felt out of control; it was her sense of responsibility, rather than her body, that weighed too much. Food was a source of power. She could dictate exactly what she put into her body. And what she didn't.

Eating is power.

I have seen a loved one give up eating for the sake of power. It wasn't a teenage girl who wanted to look like the pictures in magazines, but it *was* about control. And it was all the more heart-breaking and challenging because it was impossible to dismiss as mere vanity.

After my grandmother died, my grandfather struggled with his own health difficulties and an inability to adapt to household responsibilities alone. The realities of aging hit him hard (weakness, loss of loved ones, loneliness, isolation, boredom, a fear of being irrelevant). My grandfather reacted by losing weight. A lot of weight. This man who had lived life to the fullest, who looked and measured every inch the part of one who thrived on indulging in, enjoying, and sharing the best of food, drink, and all of the companionship and merriment that goes with it, spent his last few years fearful that if he ate a butter tart

---

1. Interview with Lionel Shriver on CBC Radio Q, Thursday, May 30, 2013.

he might "get fat." His doctor told him he was too thin. We, his closest family members, hounded him about eating more. Our concern only succeeded in feeding his resolve. He had lived a big, powerful, routinely admired, generous-to-a-fault, hub-of-the-action life, and now he felt alone, without work, health, a driver's license, or enough balance to be able to count on walking without falling.

But he could choose to eat. Or not.

If food is literally relationship—the life from outside us that forms the basis of our own life—then eating is our basic *yes* to relationship. Conversely, intentionally not eating is an effective way of reconfiguring the terms by which we are going to live. It can be a denial of relationship, the guarding of oneself against needing anything beyond the fortress of the individual self. "I am a rock, I am an island," as Simon and Garfunkel sing. It can be a means of asserting power in relationship, particularly when power is hard to come by.

Psychiatrists have noted that 50 percent of anorexia and bulimia patients report a history of sexual abuse.[2] The website AfterSilence. org, which offers support to those who have been the victims of abuse, makes the following connection around eating disorders:

> There are countless reasons why women and men (though women are still a majority) who have survived rape, sexual abuse, incest, or molestation use eating disorders as a coping mechanism. For some, developing eating disorders is a way to avoid sexuality. In other cases, an eating disorder may be a way to hide anger or frustration and seek the approval of other people. Unhealthy eating is often the symptom of a bigger problem. Since survivors often feel that they cannot show their anger and resentment directly, they may resort to unhealthy ways like starving or overeating to express on the outside what is hurting them on the inside. In addition, victims might start viewing their body as a source of shame, and an eating disorder may be used as a form of self-punishment.
>
> In stressful events like rape or molestation, the victim often feels utterly powerless, and may seek new ways to improve his or her sense

---

2. Website for *National Centre for Biotechnology Information* gets this statistic from *Psychiatry Med.* 7, no. 4 (1989): 257–67, *https://www.ncbi.nlm.nih.gov/pubmed/2602570.*

of control. Our culture and society place great emphasis on body image. Being thin is equated with maximum control. As a result, victims may start avoiding food or limiting intake to dangerous levels. By doing so, some survivors of sexual violence no longer feel powerless in their lives. Sadly, commercials, magazines, and advertisements that show unrealistic bodies can keep motivating a person to indulge in unhealthy eating behavior.[3]

Not eating then becomes an act of self-preservation, of drawing into ourselves after discovering how vulnerable we are to the hurt others can inflict, how hurtful relationships can be, or how relationships can be exploited for cruel ends. It is a mind-over-matter choice when matter (the body) is claimed as a place of pain and shame, when the lessons have all too well been taught that our bodies are deserving of cruelty, commodities to be stolen from the realm of relationship and placed on the receiving end of another's perversity, anger, or self-loathing.

Why Did I Get Sick?

Why did I get sick with an eating disorder? It's a question that comes to me more and more insistently as I remember those years of difficulty. I had loving parents. I was never abused. I was given opportunities; I was routinely encouraged to feel good about my accomplishments and to move on from failures without being destroyed. I enjoyed academics and music. I had several close friends and usually a boyfriend, even if I was never part of the popular crowd. When I encountered difficulties, my parents gave me positive tools for dealing with them. How did I come, at the age of nine, to think that my thighs compared to those of "The Fattest Woman in the World"? Where did I get the message as a twenty-something that my life would be okay if I could just drop two dress sizes? How could I have had such a healthy upbringing and yet have gotten so mired in self-loathing?

Until now, I have hidden my previous eating disorder from even the closest of my friends and family. Part of my shame and secrecy

---

3. "Eating Disorders and Sexual Violence," *After Silence*, 2007, *http://www.aftersilence.org/eating -disorders.php*.

around having had an eating disorder is connected to this feeling that I *should* have been well, that there is no good reason for anything to have been wrong with me.

Yet, I go back to Lionel Shriver's comment, "Everyone has an eating disorder." Food and love are connected through human instinct from birth. Eating, I have argued, is emotional. Thousands of years ago, the prophet Isaiah called out his people on the junk with which they were filling their lives saying, "Why do you spend your money for that which is not bread, and your labor for that which does not satisfy?" (Isa. 55:2). Human beings, across contexts and times, are susceptible to working through conflict, disappointment, and insecurity by the choices we make about what to put into our bodies. It is our default position to use our bodies as crutches, to choose unhealthy physical pleasure and the ensuing hangover of disgust and nausea that follows as a distraction from our deeper difficulties. The physical body may be part of our human story of love, but it can also be the vessel in which we deposit all that is far less than love and through which we enact the other learned stories of guilt, inadequacy, hurt, and fear.

When I was sick, I sometimes thought about the anorexic girl drowning in the sea of pillows and wondered if someday the people I loved would see that I was drowning too.

Not Drowning . . . Trying to Be Full . . .

But I wasn't drowning. Food was not my source of power in a life careening out of control. Quite the opposite. My relationship with food was about the fundamental weakness of a life centered on looking put together.

There were three or four occasions when starving felt like the solution to my desperate desire to be skinny. I never made it through even a day able to hold my resolve. The mere thought of trying to go without eating succeeded only in feeding my obsession—an all-consuming, undeniable need for food, a raging desire for the pleasure of flavor and texture and fullness of all of the sweet-sour-bitter-salty possibilities I had only begun to deny myself.

I couldn't win. I caved under the weight of this dark and living force. My attempts at control revealed how little control I had. I tried to claim power and instead gave my power away to the very thing I was trying to escape. Ultimately, my eating disorder wasn't about gaining control, it was about managing my hunger.

The Old Testament prophet Haggai declared to the Israelites, who had returned to Jerusalem from exile, "You have sown much and harvested little; you eat, but you never have enough; you drink, but you never have your fill; you clothe yourselves, but no one is warm; and you that earn wages earn wages to put them into a bag with holes" (Haggai 1:6). Mine was the insatiable, misdirected hunger of a person who suspected she was empty. Who *felt* empty. A person who had tried to fill herself, tried to appear full and complete, adequate, enough, and who, in doing so, discovered an appetite that was never satisfied. I couldn't get enough good grades, I couldn't have enough friends, I couldn't receive enough love or attract enough boys, I couldn't go to enough bars or party enough times, I didn't have enough money to buy enough clothes. Nothing alleviated the deep, resounding thud of emptiness that defined my life.

But I could conceive of any kind of food. And with a few dollars here and some occasional cooking and baking there, I made that conception of food turn into a reality. I could eat that reality. I could eat it until I was just about full. I could dream and I could savor, giving in to the sweet tease of anticipation for all that I knew I would eat later, and, when later arrived, enjoy the mouthfuls again and again and again. I was never alone. I was always accompanied: studying in my room, watching a TV show nobody else liked, surrounded by friends and family I thought were too consumed with the cares and delights of their own lives to notice me. I didn't need to be by myself if my hand was in the potato chip bag or my taste buds were being treated to a pastry. And I didn't have to own any of the consequences, as long as I could force my indulgence out of my body at some later point and wipe the slate clean in order to have my tried-and-true companion with me again the next day.

I became bulimic because I was hungry and the hunger didn't go away. I was finally lifted out of my bulimia by encountering a different sort of food.

I Am Bread

Some 80% of a loaf of bread consists of nothing more than air. But air is not nothing. . . . Air elevates our food, in every sense, raises it from the earthbound subsistence of gruel to something so fundamentally transformed as to hint at human and even divine transcendence. Surely it is no accident that Christ turned to bread to demonstrate his divinity; bread is partially inspired already, an everyday proof of the possibility of transcendence.

—Michael Pollan, *Cooked*[1]

A peasant carpenter from the backwaters of the Roman Empire blazed onto the scene setting hearts on fire, tongues to wagging, and men of power to conspiring his demise. Jesus was able to connect in an unparalleled way with people's needs and hopes. The connection, however, came at a great cost.

In the account of Jesus's life found in the Gospel of John, Jesus's identity and the risk associated with it culminated in a poignant interchange between him and his close friend Peter. Jesus had shocked his would-be followers by telling them that he was the Bread of Life. He demanded that they eat his flesh and made wild claims about the benefits of this unorthodox diet: living forever, having life within, never being hungry.

---

1. Michael Pollan, *Cooked: A Natural History of Transformation* (New York: Penguin, 2013), 249–50.

Jesus gained an abundance of new followers when he fed thousands with just a few loaves and fish. The miracle directly preceded Jesus's claiming himself as the "Bread of Life." The tangible miracle of an actual meal had attracted many, but his metaphor pushed them away. "This is too hard," most of them said. Jesus turned to the twelve who were still there and asked if they too would leave.

Peter responded, "Lord, where else can we go? You have the words of eternal life." It wasn't a resounding affirmation. Those who stayed did so with resignation, desperation even. *We have nowhere else to go.*

For Jesus, that was enough.

All four gospel accounts, along with the earliest writings of the church, indicate that Jesus equated his life with food and drink: bread and wine. He insisted on a physical, bodily relationship between his followers and himself. His disciples were told to eat his flesh, to drink his blood—to bring their deepest hunger and unquenchable thirst into their relationship with him.

We might be tempted to think that we can understand why so many followers got cold feet. It is easy to hear Jesus's chosen imagery as graphic and gory. Eating flesh, drinking blood: these commands reek of cannibalism. Even if we assume he is speaking metaphorically, his words are intimate and shocking; they break into our ultra-sanitized bubble sounding almost X-rated, and we have little frame of reference for even beginning to understand what they mean.

It is important, however, to recognize that for Jesus's Jewish listeners, his words were upsetting for different reasons than modern minds might assume. Whereas Jesus's words disturb us because we don't understand, those earliest listeners were disturbed because they understood *exactly* what he meant. Jesus was speaking into a story they understood well. His imagery was demanding, difficult, and arguably at the crux of the controversy that led to his death. Delving into the Jewish perspective is where we can gain insight into what this imagery and invitation are all about—and why people have overcome revulsion and controversy to count themselves as his followers. That perspective offers us a choice between the dominant cultural assumptions we make around food *and* a way of renewed joy in our bodies that emerges from the odd invitation to partake of body and blood.

I Am Bread—A Jewish Claim

Jesus did not need to be omniscient to know that his time was running out, that the more he challenged the systems of power of his day, and the closer to the systems of power he was when he did it, the shorter his life would be. Nevertheless, he went to Jerusalem, the holiest and most dangerous city of the Jewish world. Jesus saw the writing on the wall. He would either have to shut up, disappear, or die. On the night before his death, Jesus ate the Passover meal with his friends in an upstairs room. Leaving town would have been smarter in the face of threat, but Jesus chose the sacred act of eating and sharing in their foundational story of God liberating a band of nobody slaves from their bondage. Over the meal, Jesus told his followers that the bread and wine were his body and blood.

Within the Jewish story, the bread and wine were already evocative. Bread and wine signalled the presence of a loving God.[2] The bread hearkened back not only to the gift of manna in the wilderness, but also to the future hope of a heavenly banquet—an image of the fullness of relationship with God toward which they were journeying.

The bread and wine enjoyed during Passover were also symbols at the heart of the communal worshipping life of the Israelites throughout the rest of the year. When they were still wandering in the wilderness, they crafted the Ark of the Covenant as a portable dwelling place for God and within it they kept a piece of manna. The ark was enthroned in the first Jewish temple, but it is thought to have been stolen when the Israelites fell to the Babylonians, losing their freedom, their homeland, and their most meaningful religious symbols. When the second temple was built, it was once again at the heart of Jewish religious piety. The *Bread of the Presence* was one of three objects kept in the sacred center of the temple, the Holy of Holies. It was the priests' job to regularly offer fresh bread in this most sacred place. Wine was offered along with the bread. At their most important religious feasts—Passover, Pentecost, and Tabernacles—the priest brought the bread out for everyone to see, lifted it up, and proclaimed, "Behold God's love for you!"[3]

---

2. Brant Pitre, *Jesus and the Jewish Roots of the Eucharist* (New York: Random House, 2011), 142.
3. Ibid., 131.

Why Bread?

Bread signifies God's love because of the history that fed Jesus's people. But like all good and powerful symbols, it resonates meaningfully beyond specific knowledge of that sacred story. It connects with the universals of human experience.

- Bread was, and in many places still is, a dietary staple. In the ancient world, it was the adult equivalent of breast milk—the basic building block of a nourished life. Consider this note from Norman Wirzba: "For generations people have associated bread with food, and the availability of bread with good times and food security. In fact, the stories of successful and declining cultures are not complete without an account of the fate of their grain fields. . . . In the minds of many throughout time, without bread there simply is no life."[4]
- Bread embodies partnership. It is the result of human beings responding to the natural gift of wheat with acts of harvesting, grinding, crafting, and baking. As Wirzba goes on to note, so pivotal to the human experience is the crafting of bread from wheat that the "preparation of a loaf of bread presupposes a fairly radical transformation of our natural environment and considerable cognitive and social development."[5] Bread is a gift of God's creation, shaped by human hands.
- Despite its simplicity, and along with its identity as a basic dietary staple, bread is also delicious. Few things are as inviting and evocative a scent as freshly baking bread. As a food offered and shared, warm homemade bread elicits joy and delight.

The act of "breaking bread" is understood across human cultures as one that forges and reforges human relationships as much more than a necessary act of survival, but rather as the basis for celebration and joy, new possibility, and the nourishment of body, mind, and spirit. Perhaps Mahatma Gandhi best articulated the power of the message

---

4. Norman Wirzba, *Food and Faith: A Theology of Eating* (Cambridge: Cambridge University Press, 2011), 12.

5. Ibid., 13.

of bread, even across religious divides, when he said, "There are people in the world so hungry, that God cannot appear to them except in the form of bread."[6]

Jesus Is Bread—A Troubling Claim

Those who first heard Jesus's claim to be the Bread of Life would not have heard his "bread and body" images as cannibalism or even as some faith puzzle. For them, the equation was simple:

I am bread = I am life;

= I am God's love;

= I am nourishment/joy/partnership with God.

Jesus's words made a controversial claim. He spoke with God's authority. Ordinary bread signaled Jesus's presence, in the same way it had long signalled God's presence. Jesus's presence and God's presence were synonymous. Jesus invited his followers to feast on relationship with him with the promise that in so doing, they would experience the fulfillment of all God promised them in the Passover and the journey that followed: freedom, relationship, nourishment, and new life.

Though those first listeners may have understood his imagery, his words left them no less baffled. *How could a homeless peasant from Galilee be God's love or God's partnership or God's presence? Wasn't it wrong for a person to make such claims—especially one as humble in status and circumstance as Jesus?* They would have had to abandon all reason in order to embrace his claims. We can surely sympathize with those who found it all "too hard" to follow. The faith that Peter articulated when he said, "We have nowhere else to go," was barely enough to keep hanging on. The New Testament follows the disciples through squabbles, betrayal, and ongoing discomfort in the face of their teacher's words and actions. They ignored Jesus, ran away from him, wilfully misunderstood him, and tried to correct him. Peter himself stood outside Jesus's kangaroo trial, needing to be close, and yet, he still denied the man he couldn't seem to leave. "I do not know him!" he insisted a full three times.

6. *https://www.goodreads.com/quotes/40054-there-are-people-in-the-world-so-hungry-that-god.*

It was their stomachs that kept those early Christians following. Knowing Jesus led them to identify themselves as hungry and to believe that there might exist food that could fill them. Reluctantly, instinctively, they learned to take Jesus into their lives, to fill their bodies up with him, to understand that the life he showed them—the life in full partnership with God—existed in the flesh, and in the stomach too. They began to understand that they needed to remember that truth as often as they needed to eat. Step by step, learning The Way, they also learned to feed on the Bread of Life.

They ate the Bread and began to see the world differently. In Jesus's meal they recognized the possibility of resurrected life within an ordinary body that has walked the dusty road alongside them. They ate and their faults and failings were forgiven. They became forgiving of the faults and failings of others. They knew, finally, that God had blessed their bodies, and God had blessed the bodies of brothers and sisters to whom they had never known they were related. Their hunger led them to more than self-satisfaction and survival. It led to community, to relationship, and to a divine encounter that reshaped all human encounters. It led to joy—joy in the Body, joy in their bodies.

We Still Eat

Two thousand years later, the human stomach still provides a connecting place for this encounter, this possibility. Men and women continue to accept this odd invitation to eat, and to name this physical act as a sign of God's love. This taste of Jesus is still opening eyes to new sight. But apart from specifically Christian practice, what we collectively so desperately need to see with new eyes is food. Is it possible that the food Jesus offers can change our understanding of how we eat every meal? Can an extraordinary claim of feasting, of divine identity, of spiritual connection change the very nature of our modern relationship with food and body? To answer this, we must turn from Jesus the bread, to Jesus the guest and Jesus the host. We must look in more detail at the table fellowship so central in Jesus's ministry. We can locate challenge and possibility and new vision, both then and now, in the meal.

Habits and Healing

Sickness in the Stomach

My stomach always gave me trouble. I suffered from motion sickness as a child, which meant that I have thrown up in cars belonging to anyone I have ever cared about: parents, grandparents, friends' parents. If creating stinky scenes on family trips wasn't enough, I also have a slew of vomit stories from the school bus and amusement park rides. Only an exceedingly loyal friend would sit anywhere near me on a class trip. My puke-filled history scared off everyone except Mendi, who had a generous heart and apparently no built-in gross-out mechanism. But those were just the predictable occurrences. I was also prone to even more embarrassing spontaneous upchucking episodes. I remember no less than three times when I spewed my lunch down the aisle beside my desk to the giddy horror of my classmates. This happened as late as high school.

My mother stopped feeding me breakfast. We decided that my stomach was most unsettled in the mornings, so I gave up the supposedly most important meal of the day until I was in my early twenties. We were slower in taking other measures. I still can't imagine why, for example, I was allowed to drink grape pop or eat raspberry gummies before, or even during, any sort of travel. The vivid memories of these syrupy-sweet junk foods wreaking havoc on so many vehicles' upholstery assure me that these lessons were harder to learn.

"Why didn't you tell us you were feeling sick?" Mom would ask as we cleaned up afterward. The problem was that I always felt nauseous in the car, and I frequently felt nauseous the rest of the time. If I had told somebody every time I felt like I might throw up, I would have only succeeded in becoming Girl Crying Wolf—which, with the perspective of hindsight, might have arguably been better than Throw-Up Girl.

Misery in the Stomach

In grade five, I was miserable. I still thought of myself as a child. I didn't worry about what I wore. I wasn't interested in boys. I wore pink glasses because pink was my favorite color. My happiest times were when I was reading. I listened to show tunes, not Madonna. And I was still passionately interested in playing with dolls. I was hopelessly out of step with every other girl in my class, and I was unwilling to change in order to fit in. I don't regret being a strange kid, but I did pay for it. My classmates, both girls and boys, tormented me. I was lonely. I was weird.

I was also sick.

Whereas I would later deal with some long-learned insecurities through intentionally and forcibly making myself sick, my fifth-grade sickness manifested on a subconscious level. I hated going to school. I loved the security and ease of being at home. So I was frequently unwell. I developed a year-long cough that would get so bad at times it would end in a fit of vomiting. I stayed home for a week here and a week there with nausea and stomach pain.

I wasn't lying. I wasn't like the smart-ass kid in the movies who holds the thermometer under the nightlight so that the Mom will think they have a fever. It was no act. I felt sick. I believed I was sick. My concerned mother took me to the doctor numerous times for blood work and tests. Nothing was discernibly wrong. I was technically healthy. But my life was upsetting my stomach.

Joy in the Stomach

I am thankful that my good memories about food and my stomach outweigh these rather unpalatable ones. I most acutely remember my childhood through a collection of vivid tastes:

- Dad's sweet and spicy homemade spaghetti sauce—still my meal of choice for every one of my birthday celebrations.
- Cream of broccoli soup effortlessly crafted by my Grandma Jean—made without a recipe, and so she never made the same soup twice.
- Warm Smartie® cookies, right out of the oven, and beforehand swiping a finger through the cookie dough when Mom wasn't looking.
- Ketchup potato chips, which Mom didn't want me to eat—"*The red dye gives you cancer!*"—the salty-sweet artificial red dye taste taunted me (at a friend's house or maybe when babysitting) when I knew there was an illicit bag to be opened.
- White homemade bread crafted by my dad using my great grand-mother's recipe, served with pale homemade turkey gravy and an orange Jell-O® salad at every holiday meal. The hard butter would tear the soft bread, and my Mom would laughingly recall my great-grandmother's "apathetic housekeeper" handwritten directions for bread-making—"*Sift flour three times . . . I don't.*"
- Garlicky romaine salad. The dressing was one of the first things I learned how to make and it would make my hand stink like garlic for a day, no matter how much I scrubbed with soap. My best friend Mendi and I would eat large quantities of it then laugh at one another's bad breath, and how any boy who liked us would have to be serious enough about it to deal with the garlic as well.
- Sticky, too-sweet icing. Mendi and I sloppily blended it together out of butter, milk, icing sugar, and food dye, and then we would eat together out of the bowl.

A Lifelong Habit: What Healing Looks Like

I have enough embarrassing stories of vomit to fill an entire mem-oir. To those I can add in equal portions stories of friendship, family, belonging, joy—all processed through the stomach.

It might seem strange, given how much my unsettled stomach troubled me as a child, that I would intentionally upset my stomach when I was older. Or, perhaps in light of my having claimed eating as an inherently emotional act and an act of relationship, it might make perfect sense that a distorted understanding of self would lead me to a warped relationship with body and food. Since so many of my childhood memories, both good and bad, revolve around feelings born out in my stomach, of course I continued to physically manifest my difficulties there. Patterns are hard to break. We gravitate toward the familiar, even when the familiar is decidedly unpleasant.

The point is that my eating disorder was not just a few months of my life, or even a year or two of self-destructive behavior. I fell back into habits I had developed long before I was conscious that I was making decisions. At the same time, I was forming a new habit of receiving food as the gift that it is. It took a long time to be able to accept this gift, to see my love of food as something other than a narcotic, a liability, or a weakness.

I sometimes think about Bartimaeus, that character in the gospels whose blindness led him to holler to Jesus for healing. My night of cake and prayer and purging brought me a special kinship with him. His encounter became my encounter.

Bartimaeus got what he wanted. He was blind and then he could see. Did he sometimes forget he was once blind? Did his vision occasionally cloud and narrow? Years down the road, did he continue to find new possibilities of sight? Did the challenges of life wear away at his gratitude? At some point illness or catastrophe or old age overtook him. He might have been healed, but he was still mortal. He received no exemption from weakness and frailty and death.

Men and women in the pages of the gospel story encounter Jesus and receive mobility, forgiveness, cleansing, and deliverance from demons. The story of Jesus continues on, but we rarely hear again from the ones he made well and left behind. If Jesus's disciples are any measure, if the consistent witness of the saints over the centuries can be trusted, then the healing that one receives is lived out in an entirely human way—with setbacks and new insights, fresh mistakes, limited perspectives, and also an unfolding wisdom as that healing takes root in an individual life.

I shared my story of bulimia and healing with a friend of mine, who in turn asked me if you could be cured of bulimia. Alcoholics are taught that they are always in recovery and that recovery happens one day at a time. "Can you actually have an eating disorder in the past?" she wondered. It's a good question. I can only answer from my own experience.

I don't make myself throw up anymore. I haven't since that night of prayer and vomit. But I wasn't actively bulimic when that happened. It had been over three years since I had stuck my fingers down my throat. Before that night, however, I still lived with an eating disorder. I was miserable in my body and distressed by the food I put into it. So what changed? What old life was suddenly, noticeably gone?

The obsessions lifted. That might not sound like a lot, but for anyone who has been caught in a mind frame that relentlessly repeats, you will know how extraordinary this is. My body and mind used to be split into warring factions. I had been tortured in my relationship with food and my body for as long as I could remember. I fixated on any comment about the size of my stomach, references to my being bigger than my smaller friends, and the thoughtless warnings of "*be careful eating that, you'll get fat.*"

And then suddenly the weapons were laid down and a new peace was possible. Like Bartimaeus, my lifelong pattern of blindness ended. I no longer fight the daily battle between food cravings and self-loathing, between some mythical picture of happiness and fulfillment and the twenty pounds of body fat I need to lose to attain it. I no longer go to bed each night planning what I will eat the next day, only to come to the end of that day brutally disappointed in myself for all of the ways I broke down and gave in. I have some graciously granted acceptance of my own body, and in turn I have been released of much of the constant dissatisfaction that once consumed me and made be believe I wasn't good enough.

Along with my changed mindset has come a stable, healthy body weight. Most amazingly, I am free to enjoy food. I can eat and savor the flavor and give thanks for the joy and fellowship the gift of food brings to my life without toppling back into the addiction where I used food to anaesthetize feelings and projected onto it all of my insecurities and failures. I know now that the fixations were from inside, but I was coddled in those fixations from the comments and the learned behaviors of dieting and body dissatisfaction at play outside and around me, related not to any valid criticism of me or my body, but to a deep societal dis-ease with food and bodies.

The obsessions I lived with my whole life lifted. That is the gift. I can now honestly say that somehow, miraculously, I no longer have an eating disorder.

Healed, But Very Human

I don't want to misrepresent myself. The healing I've experienced, as profound as it has felt to me, is still lived out in an entirely human way. I still feel fat some days. I have moments of wondering why my thighs are so big and if that's what other people see as my most glaringly obvious feature too. Sometimes I eat too much and I feel awful afterward.

In response to these little slips I have learned practices that help me stay on track. One night I went to sleep praying at the feet of Jesus that he would make me better. My life was different after that. I received healing. But healing is not just a gift; it is also a responsibility. I can tell you that my own continued healing requires that I stay close to the one who gave me new life. I didn't figure out these practices myself: I learned them.

I am still learning them.

You Are How You Eat

learned many healthy lessons about food and eating from my family. Sunday night dinners provided the backbone of what my parents believed, of the life they shared with us through the gift of food.

The meal would begin late in the afternoon with friends arriving. We had a core group of guests—Nancy, Marg, sometimes Talph, and oftentimes the priest from our church and his family—who by virtue of sharing almost weekly in this feast together, became "family by choice." The occasion was elevated slightly if grandparents happened to be there, in which case we would also get a game of cards going during the afternoon. There must have been wine, although I don't remember it being a key component of the gathering, and there were simple snacks put out to munch as we discussed the week's events. Often there were extra friends around our table because my parents made it clear that the supper invitation was ours to share too.

The fare was simple but tasty: a roast, vegetable, salad, potatoes, gravy, and dessert. There was always enough for at least one dinner of leftovers through the week, so Sunday night meals were both celebratory and practical. Everything was homemade. Our dining room table was large, and it was my job to hold one end in place while my Mom wrestled the expansion boards to extend the table. We had a beautiful crocheted tablecloth that she loved to use on the more special occasions. It took my grandmother months to make, and I remember how pleased Mom was when Grandma gave it to her one Christmas. I thought it a risky thing to use in the presence of greasy gravy and tipsy beverages, but the fact that tablecloths would be spilled on has never been a barrier for my mother using them. The conversations were equal parts serious and silly. Religion and politics, those two supposedly most taboo subjects, got the most airtime. However, Mom put an end to any "bathroom talk" or descriptions of illness or injury. "We don't need to talk about that at the supper table," she will say.

Though I got mired in destructive thoughts and habits about food, these family meals—and all of the weekday meals that were also structured around words of gratitude, open invitations, and balanced homemade food—were the counterpoint. I pray that the blessing of sharing in my parents' meals will feature in my family's life for many more years. I aspire to create a similar table of laughter, welcome, and flavor in my own home.

✿ ✿ ✿

You are what you eat. By now, it is an overused colloquialism. Yet, in both literal and poetic ways, Christianity claims that what we eat forms who we are. At the heart of the practice of Eucharist (also referred to as "Communion" or "The Lord's Supper" in other denominational traditions), we share the broken bread in Jesus's name that "he might dwell in us, and we in him."

But before Jesus taught "You are what you eat," he taught "You are *how* you eat." How you eat communicates much about what you value, who you value, and indeed who you are.

Consider the person eating a Double Big Mac, large fries, and a Diet Coke. Picture that person eating in their car on the way from one obligation to another. I might, if feeling judgmental, draw certain conclusions. For example, they look lonely and busy. Their life appears to be structured in a way that makes convenience a higher priority than health. I could surmise that this person is probably not an environmentalist, a farmer, or the owner of a small local business. The diet could indicate a tension around eating: they are opting for a chemical-laden beverage for a highly suspect method of calorie control while continuing to fill their body with calorie-excessive, nutritionally poor junk food. Their particular food choices might even signal illness. Diet soda might mean they are one of many North Americans who now suffer from diabetes. Double Big Macs and large fries could tell me they have become diabetic mostly through bad eating choices.

Am I right in my conclusions? Maybe not. Are these fair assumptions to be making about an individual I do not know? No. Have I ever gone through the McDonald's drive-thru? Yes, and I am someone who would name the environment, my family, and my health as things I care about, even if I am not perfect in how I live out these priorities. This person who has unwittingly become my example could very well be acting out a quick-fix anomaly in a life highly committed to community, family, and health. They were in a rush and needed something to eat, fast.

But conclusions that are unfair to draw in the case of one individual become more justifiable when we broaden the scope and look at cultural patterns. Collectively, we rely on commercially prepared food and eat in our cars more and more frequently—and this is producing not only dire health consequences for us, but also creating a crisis in our oceans and in our landfills because of the single-use plastics wrapping up all of our convenience food. Collectively, we throw out almost half of the food that we buy—and we do this while food bank use escalates across North America and food insecurity accelerates around the globe. Collectively, our increasing appetite for cheap meat and nonseasonal produce all year round means that we see little connection between the food we eat and the animals, farmlands, and laborers who make it possible.

Whereas our observation of the person eating takeout in their car is just a best guess of what they value, our broader cultural patterns paint a picture of what we, as a society, have chosen to prioritize.

We are *how* we eat. Jesus understood that. It is no wonder then that Jesus could be found, throughout his ministry, at the dinner table. The meals he shared provoked controversy and consternation and sent a clear message about how Jesus was making real the preposterous proclamation that *the kingdom of God has drawn near.* Jesus used food and table fellowship to expose the value systems of his day and, in so doing, to inaugurate a whole new world.

Jesus's Response to Exclusion

Jesus lived in a world that clearly defined "who is in" and "who is out." It was a culture with strict purity codes. Social cues were easy to read because people were defined by stratified categories of worth. Life was challenging and unjust, but at least people knew where they stood. Political and religious leaders maintained power by controlling the rules for the basic act of eating. Overall, people were willing to follow the rules. In exchange, they received a sense of stability and security in the midst of a volatile world. Sharing a meal meant that the people involved were of the same religion, followed the same dietary restrictions, and were on the same economic strata of society. Those who did not adhere to society's codes ate alone.

Jesus ate with sinners and outcasts. He received a drink of water from a woman of a different religion. He accepted an invitation to dine with a tax collector. He welcomed a prostitute into the middle of a dinner gathering. The religious elite of his day showed signs, at first, of a willingness to cozy-up to Jesus, to claim him as one of their own and use his obvious gifts for their own ends. But he kept letting in the riff-raff, and therefore they had to turn on him. He contradicted the commonly held belief that using power to manage people was God's will. Instead, Jesus bore witness to the God who broke down barriers; the God who revealed the truth that everyone is related to one another, bound to one another—even to those we "can't stomach." God's mission was healing and forgiveness and community, not carefully managed alienation.

Jesus's choice of eating companions clearly signaled an unbridgeable chasm between the values of the day and the values of the realm he proclaimed. In reaction, the religious leadership believed they had no option but to plot Jesus's demise.

Jesus's Response to Scarcity

Jesus lived in a world of "not enough." Scarcity breeds starvation, want, and need, which in turn produce fear and the survival instinct—*looking after our own*. As Jesus roamed the Galilean countryside, he saw the desperate circumstances in which his people lived. Rome raised taxes, families lived on less and less, more people succumbed to the pressures of debt, and the majority of people were one day's wage away from gnawing hunger.

In Jesus's most widely reported miracle, he ended a day of teaching in the countryside with a remarkable feast. The gospels claimed that four or five thousand men, plus women and children, were stranded without food. They had been so anxious to feast on Jesus's words that their rumbling stomachs caught them by surprise.

Jesus fed the thousands with a few loaves and fishes, providing food enough that everyone ate until full; more than that, everyone ate until there were baskets of leftovers collected at the end. Jesus claimed a different reality from scarcity. There was enough. There was more than enough. God had blessed them with an abundance of good gifts. The kingdom of God looked like a world where people were fed, where everyone discovered they had something to share and to receive.

Jesus's Response to Fear

Jesus sat at table with his friends on a dark night in a darkening world. In those defining hours of Jesus's life—his last words, his last actions, his final song—there was a meal. Jesus had arrived in Jerusalem the Sunday before. Jerusalem was the center of his people's power. Pilgrims from all over Judea had been pouring into the city to celebrate the Passover. In his actions and his teachings throughout the week, Jesus put himself at odds with both Rome and his own people's leadership who were desperately trying to maintain stability within a fractured and oppressive system. Jesus knew his time was running out, that his words and actions would not go unchallenged, and that all of those who had been threatened by the new world he proclaimed and the God he made so real were about to close in on him.

Jesus did not run. He ate.

Jesus gave thanks, broke bread, poured wine. He said strange words of remembrance, new life, covenant, and forgiveness. In John's gospel, the meal is accompanied by an action. Jesus gave the new commandment of love to his disciples and then enacted it by washing their feet. Jesus lived in a world where peace was imposed through military power, where might was always right, where people were kept quiet and cooperative by the institutionalization of fear. If Jesus and his disciples knew what was good for them, they would have hit the road.

Instead, they ate.

Jesus found courage to tell the truth at that table. To stand his ground. To bear witness. To proclaim that, in the end, God would make good on the promise that their simple and vulnerable acts of friendship and thanksgiving and resistance had world-changing power.

"*This is my body. This is my blood.*"

Jesus's Response to Isolation: New Creation

Cementing the promise that in the ordinary elements of bread and wine we experience Jesus as living, the risen Christ kept showing up just in time to eat—fish in a locked room, a sunrise barbeque on the beach, broken bread in Emmaus. In these meals the disciples, one by one, step by step, became convinced that the new life Jesus offered was real. Through the sharing of food, they began to experience themselves as forgiven, healed, enlivened, and loved. In the four-fold practice enacted in Jesus's life—blessing, breaking, sharing, sending—the old order of death and despair that defined daily life and the values embodied in its eating practices were not merely destroyed, but also revealed as having never been real.

Jesus's life culminated in resurrection—the new creation. Jesus made it clear that this new creation ate differently. And in eating differently, Jesus's followers not only saw but began to *taste* the truth and power and life at the center of Jesus's prayer and proclamation—a renewed people and a reclaimed world.

Exclusion, Scarcity, Fear, and Isolation Today

Exclusion, scarcity, fear, and isolation remain as powerful forces at work in our world today. They fuel the food industry, which tells us that our bodies are unrelated to other bodies, deserving of our obsessive attention but not our respect. These forces play out in different ways today than in Jesus's time, and yet they are just as powerful now as they were then.

Exclusion—Young bodies are sexualized, idolized, and manipulated. Celebrity bodies are worshipped, critiqued, and consumed. Old bodies are abused, ridiculed, and forgotten. Poor bodies are blamed, exploited, and ignored. Animal bodies are used for pets and protein.

Scarcity—Our reliance on cheap and junky food at the expense of food economies that perpetuate prosperity or environmental responsibility reveals an uncritical deeply held belief in scarcity. We don't have enough time. We don't have enough energy. We don't have enough money. So we eat hastily, thoughtlessly in our cars, while multitasking at our desks, or on our phones. We value quantity over quality and survival over community. Meanwhile the discrepancy between the overfed and the starving is a blight on our global civilization.

Fear—Our bodies can break down or bloat up, our bodies can hurt and get fat and release the memories of who we are. Our bodies will die. And yet the multitude of face creams and diets marketed to us to feed an obsession with attaining a perfect body actually belies a barely concealed fear of the vulnerability of being mortal, as well as the consciousness to know it.

Isolation—We are taught that what we put into our bodies has no bearing on the people or ecosystems around us. We are not part of a chain, a system, a life. Furthermore, the same disconnection we so wholeheartedly believe about how our bodies exist in relationship with the world is also lived out as disconnection and alienation within the individual self. People are hyperconnected through Google and social media, and yet many have never felt more alone.[1]

---

1. "Study after study finds that people of all ages feel lonelier and more isolated. In 2008, a landmark study conducted by the University of Chicago discovered that one-in-five Americans often felt lonely. And according to the AARP, in 2010, two-in-five seniors often felt the pain of being alone, up from 20 percent in the '80s. Meanwhile, in the U.K., the Mental Health Foundation reported that nearly three-in-five young adults aged 18 to 34, despite all their social networking, admitted to feeling isolated and disconnected often or all the time." (Kat Ascharya, "How Social Media Is Making Us Lonelier," *Modern Health*, posted on 2machines.com.)

Jesus's Response Today

I know what it is to be reconfigured. You may relate to parts of my story, or my sharing might invite you to a deeper and more considered reflection of your own relationship with your body and the food you put into it. In our quest for health and healing in our attitudes toward food and eating, the next step is to get practical. Christianity is a practical faith grounded in bodily existence. Where do God's alternatives connect with practice? How can these practices change our attitudes and our health? How is this new way of life related to the radical claim that we should follow our stomachs and eat the body of Christ? If we truly are *how* we eat, then how could we eat in order to reconfigure not just ourselves, but our world?

Part two takes us into the heart of these questions. I can't give you a formula that will lead to a visceral experience of prayer like the one I received, but I can share the choices, the perspective, the community, and the relationships that now keep me well. I can take us from the Jesus who responded through table fellowship to the isolation, exclusion, scarcity, and fear of his first-century companions to the eating practices that can offer a similar response to our distorted relationship with food today. These Jesus practices form the Living Diet—a diet of feasting, fasting, moving, speaking, sharing, hungering, praying, worshipping, connecting, remembering, storytelling, and even dying. This diet re-creates us for partnership: God's creation shaped by our human hands, offered to God in thanksgiving, returned by God to us as blessing. In that partnership, we discover the possibility of a world where all are fed, where we understand "enough," where each knows and receives what they actually need. Most importantly, this diet takes seriously our hungriest questions—*Do I have enough? Am I enough?*—and feeds us with the new possibility of what our lives are for.

part
2

The Diet

Becoming Real

// | don't go to church anymore," a woman informed me as we were
       | introduced by a mutual friend. Because of my line of work, peo-
       | ple often feel that they have to tell me the status of their faith
life. She continued, "It's all about making people feel guilty, and I just
don't need that."

This is a common complaint. Faith communities have gar-
nered a reputation for dishing out helpings of guilt. Her accusa-
tory tone and closed body language suggested she wasn't looking
for a response, but I would have liked to have pointed out that human
beings need no help from the church to feel guilty. "If you're not feeling guilty about something as a new mother," a new-mother-friend of
mine once said to me, "you're doing something wrong." She might
have made the same observation about our eating, our work, our
downtime, our spending habits, our need to wear daily sunscreen,
or our cell phone use. If we're not feeling guilty about whatever it is
we may or may not be doing, we're probably just not thinking about
it enough.

The church doesn't need to make us feel guilty. We are good at feeling guilty all by ourselves. Many have walked away from the church's
so-called version of guilt only to find themselves still saddled with the
messages of inadequacy and failure they get everywhere else.

The Cleanse: The New Ritual Purification

> If you called it "Celebrity Crank Diet" it would not catch on. But calling it "A Cleanse" dignifies it. It speaks to this idea of ritual cleansing present in just about all of the great religions of the world. I think that part of its appeal is this wish to not be these secular, overprivileged, overfed characters that many of us are, but to cleanse ourselves to be something higher, purer, more ascetic, more in touch with our souls, and less with our bodies.
>
> —Katherine Ashenburg, author of *The Dirt on Clean*[1]

In the book *Is Gwyneth Paltrow Wrong about Everything?*, Professor Timothy Caulfield examines a popular dietary fad: the cleanse. Although he concludes that there is no research to support the health claims made by these dietary cleanses, Caulfield remains sympathetic to the cultural and even religious reasons why they have become so appealing.[2]

Caulfield argues that the use of semireligious language is intentional and part of what makes these radical cleanses intuitively appealing. People gravitate toward a solution for addressing a particularly insidious version of guilt. Holiday feasting or normal patterns of indulgence, of eating and drinking with family and friends, is recast as sinful. Where we might have once looked to religion to offer absolution for our "sins," now a fancy celebrity cleanse is marketed to us instead: we can repent from bad eating behavior and restart our systems, making ourselves clean again. Religious piety holds very little clout in our society anymore, but *dietary* piety is seen as good, noble, admirable. It is a way of asserting power over our bodies, and therefore over the world around us. Cleanses are marketed as a "system restart," "a purification," or a chance to "get the trash out of your colon."

That human impulse to feel guilty or even unclean is as strong as ever, even with the weakened hold organized religion has on our collective psyche. And there are those who will manipulate that guilty impulse toward their own benefit. Whether in particular versions of church, or particular versions of dieting, we can find the package that

---

1. Interview on CBC Radio, *Q Arts & Culture Show*, January 4, 2016.

2. Ibid.

promises to make us clean again. We turn our lives—whether on the spiritual plane or the physical one—into battlegrounds where our baser impulses toward indulgence and frivolity are brought to heel by that someone or something setting up the parameters within which we are allowed to count ourselves purified.

The New Religion: Modern-Day Food Culture

Geneen Roth quotes some astounding statistics in the beginning of her book *Women, Food and God*:

> In an April 2007 UCLA study of the effectiveness of dieting, researchers found that one of the best predictors of weight gain was having lost weight on a diet at some point during the years before the study started. Among those who were followed for fewer than two years, 83 percent gained back more weight than they had lost. Another study found that people who went on diets were worse off than people who didn't.[3]

Cleanses, like the culture of dieting itself, are masters in creating the conditions for failure. They allow for a radical sense of purification, results are quick and noticeable, but ultimately the practices are unsustainable; weight lost is quickly weight regained. They provide an appealing, but very temporary, sense of relief from the extra psychological and physical weight we are carrying, and they require that we keep cycling back into taking up that burden again, and with it all of the disappointment and guilt we've learned to feel about our bodies.

Food is the new religion in North America. We have different denominations, each claiming their own particular scriptures. There are varying levels of piety and purity and adherence. We judge who is in and who is out based on which practices are adopted and how well. Our media gather us around the shared practices of both worshipping and hating the body. We turn the gift of food, meant to support and nourish us, into a system of rules and regulations, with guilt as the sheepdog herding us constantly into the pen of complacency.

---

3. Geneen Roth, *Women, Food, and God: An Unexpected Path to Almost Everything* (New York: Simon & Schuster, 2010), 29.

What if our food choices weren't about becoming clean and beautiful and having great skin? What if our eating led us to become more vulnerable and honest with one another and the world around us? To be okay with our shabbiness and frailty? To see real life, real bodies—our own included—as beautiful?

Clean? Or Real . . . ?

"The glory of God is the human being fully alive."

—Irenaeus, second century

In the Christian tradition, baptism is strongly associated with repentance and forgiveness. Water symbolizes cleaning, purification, washing something dirty away. The same premise that makes a Gwyneth Paltrow cleanse so intuitively appealing is present in that ancient language and symbolism used around baptism: a system reset, a starting over, a cleansing, a purification. Baptism is a one-time rite, but Christians are encouraged to remember and renew our baptism regularly. In some Christian traditions, worship starts with the Asperges—the blessing of water, sprinkling it on the congregation—"Purge me with hyssop, and I shall be clean; wash me, and I shall be whiter than snow" (Ps. 51:7).

But if we look to the story of Jesus's own baptism, we find another possibility in how we might understand this central Christian ritual. All four gospels are consistent in seeing Jesus's baptism as a defining moment, launching him from obscurity as an unknown peasant carpenter into a highly controversial and magnetic public ministry. And yet, when Jesus emerged from his full-body plunge by John into the Jordan River, it was not a message of purification that he received. "You are my beloved son," a voice from heaven thundered. "With you I am well pleased." Jesus had, as yet, done nothing in particular to please God. He had not embraced his identity as Messiah in any obvious way. He had not proven himself; he had not met expectations; he had not lived a life that was noteworthy or extraordinary. But God loved him. God embraced him as a beloved child.

In contrast to that impulse toward purification, the transformative love offered by God to Jesus connects me to another story. I heard it first when my second-grade teacher read it to my class. Though it was not one of the formative books of my childhood, I have been moved as an adult to become reacquainted with the story and to read it in turn to my own children. I connect it now to Jesus's baptism, not because of the details of the baptism story itself, but because I know what happened once Jesus emerged from the water. I know the demons and dirt, the terror and betrayal and the unclean hope that greeted Jesus as his baptism launched him into his new public role. *The Velveteen Rabbit* by Margery Williams is about Rabbit, a stuffed animal whose life is inextricably tied to the boy who owns him. It is about how Rabbit can potentially be shaped by the possibility of love:

> "What is REAL?" asked the Rabbit one day, when they were lying side by side near the nursery fender, before Nana came to tidy the room. "Does it mean having things that buzz inside you and a stick-out handle?"
>
> "Real isn't how you are made," said the Skin Horse. "It's a thing that happens to you. When a child loves you for a long, long time, not just to play with, but REALLY loves you, then you become Real."
>
> "Does it hurt?" asked the Rabbit.
>
> "Sometimes," said the Skin Horse, for he was always truthful. "When you are Real you don't mind being hurt."
>
> "Does it happen all at once, like being wound up," he asked, "or bit by bit?"
>
> "It doesn't happen all at once," said the Skin Horse. "You become. It takes a long time. That's why it doesn't happen often to people who break easily, or have sharp edges, or who have to be carefully kept. Generally, by the time you are Real, most of your hair has been loved off, and your eyes drop out and you get all loose in the joints and very shabby. But these things don't matter at all, because once you are Real you can't be ugly, except to people who don't understand."[4]

There is nothing in Jesus's story that suggests he sought baptism in order to be cleansed. What he needed was to become. He needed

---

4. Margery Williams, *The Velveteen Rabbit* (New York: Bantam Doubleday Dell Publishing Group, 1922), 5–8.

to become able to see that he, a humble carpenter from Galilee, could bear God's Light. He needed to become capable of being hurt, and to know that being hurt would not destroy him. He needed to become an offering, surrendering himself and trusting he would not lose himself in letting go.

He needed to become the relationship revealed in those unearned words of love spoken to him after his immersion in the Jordan. And the only way to become that relationship was to recognize and name the myriad of characters he would meet on the dusty road as his family, though many of them were not obviously connected to him at all. The love that took him into dark territory and bound him in relationship was the witness Jesus bore to the world as a human being becoming real.

Bread of Life

Jesus claimed he was the Bread of Life: he was the embodiment of God's love. And he invited his followers to be nourished by him. What does it mean to be nourished by Jesus? To fill our lives with him? To be fed by Christ? Jesus's words were offered, first, as a response to the hunger he saw in his followers.

Jesus understands that our hunger can lead us to settle for junk, which leads to guilt about the junk, and then a search for that junk-free fresh start and the squeaky clean body that points to a purified soul. Jesus's claim to be the Bread of Life invites us instead to see that our hunger can lead us to community, relationship, and joy. He calls us to see that we gravitate toward these messages of guilt because the guilt is an expression of the powerlessness of living lives that are so tainted by the world around us. Jesus's voice of love beckons us into the waters, to name us as beloved, even as we feel muddled about in the mess around and within us. As we are nourished by his love, we are able to embrace the awkward beauty of human life, and in doing so, we can become not pure, but connected; not clean, but real.

We are *how* we eat. Jesus teaches us to eat differently, and therefore to live differently—to *be* differently. Or maybe, more accurately, Jesus teaches us how to become more fully ourselves.

A New Diet, A Living Diet

Before the word "diet" meant anything else, before it was attached to weight loss and celebrities and cleanses and best-selling books and the products to go with them, it simply meant "way of life," or "manner of living." If I were trying to emulate Gwyneth Paltrow, I would have rules and recipes for you to follow, and you would want to follow them because of the health, vitality, youth, and weight loss that I would promise, accompanied by some impressive formulas (counting carbs, calories, vitamins, and fiber portions) that would make it sound like food and bodies can be controlled by math.

I'm not going to do any of that. Instead, I'm going to offer some stories that respond to the questions I have begun to pose: *What does it look like to eat the Bread of Life? If we are **how** we eat, how do we eat in order to become more fully alive? How do we eat to become more real?* I have found the most compelling understanding of "real" by paying attention to Jesus, the love spoken at his baptism, and the way he then lived that love in the world. Rather than formulas, I see new patterns of relationship for our food, our bodies, and the world that isn't just around us, but is in us. These stories are mine, my friends', my family's, and my faith community's, and they compose the backbone of what I call the Living Diet. The diet, or *way of living*, that emerges from these stories is grounded in experience and is shared with others who have learned the truth that "thin" is not the same as being alive.

I have grouped these stories into explorations of thanksgiving and hunger, feasting and fasting, moving and speaking, reconnecting body and world, worshipping and dying. And there is even an important place for some cake along the way!

In contrast to the fad and celebrity diets out there, and in homage to the gentleness with which the Christian life is meant to be adopted ("Take my yoke upon you . . . for I am gentle" [Matt. 11:29]), the Living Diet offers a range of options that can be incorporated by families and singles, people of varying economic means and different amounts of time to commit to change. Because it is ultimately about a shift in attitude, rather than a prescription for what to eat and not eat, and because even small steps in that shift can create extraordinary results, I assume that the Living Diet is best and most reasonably adopted in part rather than in whole, and I trust too that you will discern which parts speak to you.

I don't have rules or recipes. Friends of mine will be relieved to know that I'm not going to use this book as a platform for promoting kale as a dietary staple. I do, however, offer a wild promise. It is not some magical key that will unlock the fountain of youth or a swimsuit-ready body. I promise instead that in surrendering to the reality of who we really are and how our lives are thoroughly mixed up in the world around us, we can change our eating habits into ones that bring blessing, freedom, and joy. I promise that the Living Diet will allow us not to be purer and more in control, but rather to become more real.

Gratitude—A Eucharistic Life

t is common practice for our Canadian Indigenous communities to
engage in water ceremonies, gathering at the community's source of
water and speaking or singing words of blessing and thanksgiving.
In 2007, the First Nations' community of Rama blessed water from a
particularly polluted and troubled part of our Ontario waterways. The
Rama tell of how government researchers took pH readings before and
after the ceremony as part of their regular monitoring schedule. The
reading after the blessing showed a dramatic drop in acidity—a temporary neutralizing of the pollution.[1]

A 1997 study by Dr. Masaru Emoto in Japan examined the microscopic structure of water molecules in response to different sorts of
feelings and words:

> Dr. Masaru Emoto discovered that crystals formed in frozen water
> reveal changes when specific, concentrated thoughts are directed toward
> them. He found that water from clear springs and water that has been
> exposed to loving words shows brilliant, complex, and colorful snow-
> flake patterns. In contrast, polluted water, or water exposed to negative
> thoughts, forms incomplete, asymmetrical patterns with dull colors.[2]

1. A story shared in a sermon on February 3, 2013, at St. David's Anglican-Lutheran Church,
Orillia, by Christine Douglas, a member of the Rama First Nations' community.

2. Dr. Masaru Emoto's work is featured in the documentary *What the Bleep Do We Know!?*
More information can be found at *https://whatthebleep.com/water-crystals/*.

I don't know how these accounts stand up to scientific scrutiny. "It might be more of an art project than science," my friend Katherine commented about the water molecule images. Being art, of course, doesn't make it less true. As the leader of a faith community, I hear and see many stories of how the physical world is altered by the words and prayers we choose to speak over it. The truth held up in the Rama story and in the crystalline images is that our words, our intentions, and our attitudes impact the physical world around us.

Boiled rice, as one basic food example, is over 70 percent water. An adult human body is 57 to 60 percent water. We can imagine our food and our bodies on a molecular level looking either crystalline or cloudy, depending on the words we choose to describe ourselves and the food we consume. I wonder what the damage looked like on a molecular level during those years that I felt such animosity toward my body. What can I make of the grace bestowed on me that, despite those years of warfare, my body returned my animosity by participating in the most awe-inspiring experiences of childbirth and breastfeeding?

That's a personal question. There are collective questions to raise as well. What effect does our attitude toward food really have on how our bodies then digest it? How does our guilty angst or our entitled apathy inform the molecular structure of the food we eat? How do simple acts of thanksgiving or blessing over our food change what we are eating?

The Problem

Common dieting advice says, "Don't be afraid to leave your plate unfinished." It sounds reasonable, and I understand the rationale. Portion sizes have increased. Don't mindlessly overeat just because the food is there. Whereas I have respect for any method that takes into account how my body actually feels, the casual wastefulness suggested by this advice bothers me as someone whose natural inclination is toward economy and frugality. More importantly, the attitude that eating is an individual activity and that food is only about me and my needs is representative of our warped North American difficulty with eating.

Every sphere of the food industry encourages us to think about food as a cheap and disposable resource for our own personal pleasure,

reward, indulgence, or weakness. From the overpackaging of products, to the garbage bags behind bakeries full of "day-old bread," to the
seemingly reasonable advice to leave food on our plates when we feel
that we are full, we hold an unchallenged, and therefore casual, attitude
of wastefulness toward food.

Eucharist

> While they were eating, Jesus took a loaf of bread, and after
> blessing it he broke it, gave it to the disciples, and said, "Take,
> eat; this is my body." (Matt. 26:26)

Christian worship offers food: metaphysical, spiritual food, but ultimately, literal food as well. There is a meal at the heart of our worship.
Although church is often assumed to be about something special, a step
outside of our normal, everyday lives, at the center of our regular worshipping life is a remarkably normal, everyday act. And we often miss
it. For long-time churchgoers, worship can become so rote and familiar that we fail to see what we are actually doing. On the other hand,
for new or nonchurchgoers, worship may seem like a club for insiders,
disconnected from any non-church-related knowledge and experience.

In fact, Christian worship is centered fully in the stuff of life. The
earliest band of Jesus's followers formed themselves into the community of the church through the liturgy of eating. And as this pattern of
worship and formation developed, it attracted a name that doesn't just
describe the ritual and praise of the church coming together, but also
extends to offer a possibility for everyday household life.

The regular pattern of Christian worship is called Eucharist, which
means "thanksgiving." This primary form of praise is about recognizing, receiving, and practicing gratitude and generosity. The Eucharistic
Prayer is the culmination of worship and is modeled after Jewish table
prayers of blessing. It is the part of the service when the bread and
the wine are offered at the altar—God's table—and we recount how
God has been revealed to us in creation, in the biblical witness, and
in Jesus. We remember specifically Jesus's final night before his death
and the meal he shared with his closest followers. But the many other
meals that illuminated his life and ministry are also referenced: eating

with outsiders and sinners, feeding thousands with a few loaves and fish, and resurrection accounts where Jesus's new life is recognized "in the breaking of the bread." We pray that God's Spirit will reveal Jesus's presence to *us* through the bread and the wine. We do not just remember the meals, we ask that they become part of our lives, forming us in the same patterns of healing, compassion, forgiveness, and courage.

Ablutions

In my Anglican/Episcopal tradition, there are certain rituals that take place after the Eucharist. The rest of the bread and wine are consumed. The priest, or one of the servers, might do this on their own. If there is a lot left over, others may be called to help eat and drink. Extra wine can be poured down a sink-like shaft, which goes directly to the ground instead of feeding into the regular sewer system. What can seem like fussy rituals follow the focused eating of the leftovers. The plate that was used for the bread is held over the empty chalice. Water is poured over the plate, collecting both the water and any extra crumbs into the chalice. The water is swished around to remove the legs of wine that may have gathered on its sides. Someone, often the priest, is tasked with drinking the somewhat unpalatable concoction of dregs. Further rinsing and swishing is performed as needed. And in some congregations, this ritual is extended. First, the cup is rinsed with extra wine, then with water and crumbs, then with more water. The small white linen used for wiping the chalice during Communion, called the purificator, is used to wipe the plate and chalice and is placed into the chalice when all is done. Altar guild members follow specific instructions for washing the linens so that any stains of wine or any stray crumbs are removed with an attention to where those stains and crumbs are going. No visible speck is to be ignored or tossed aside. Any unconsumed bread or wine is placed in a small cupboard, called an ombrey, or, in fancier churches, into a tabernacle. A light is kept lit nearby. You might see the faithful bowing down, even genuflecting, before the reserved sacrament. When all of this is done well, a gentle care is visible. It is more than just going through the motions of cleaning up. Thoughtfulness and love are the guiding principles.

It isn't always done well. It can get fussy. People have been known to become paranoid or rude over the ways in which the extra bread and wine are treated. I have been snapped at a few times in my training over missing some minute detail or not being sufficiently reverent while eating the leftovers. If this is Jesus's body and blood, we can't waste, lose, or mistreat any of it. On the other hand, I have heard more laid-back priests wisecrack, "If Jesus can get into the bread, I'm sure he can get out again."

Although these rituals can be written off as mysterious and unnecessary, there is also something about these actions worth noting. When we celebrate communion at God's table, there are a number of things that we recognize as happening to the bread and wine we share together at that meal:

- The bread and wine are *offered*. The gifts we bring forward from our community were first gifts given to us by God; they are made from wheat and grape, gifts of God's creation, and shaped by human hands into food and drink. By virtue of participating in God's creation, they are already holy. They are important symbols of our own lives—*already* in partnership with God, *already* the recipients of God's good gifts, whether we appreciate them or not.

- The bread and wine are *consecrated*. This means we intentionally ask the blessing of God's Spirit on this bread and wine so that they may be revealed as holy *to us*. When we intentionally participate in seeing something as holy, we believe that the thing that we have asked God to bless is consecrated.

- The bread is *broken*, the wine *poured*. The bread and wine, *shared* together, become part of how we experience our belief that Jesus lives. Breaking bread with people—people who were hungry, alone, scared, isolated, guilty, broken, as well as people who were joyful, grateful, healed—was such a big part of Jesus's life and witness that the church from the earliest times has broken bread and shared wine in order to tangibly and physically experience Jesus's presence. And so we say these strange and haunting words about the bread—"The body of Christ"—and about the wine—"The blood of Christ." We share the bread and wine together, and we become part of how those words are true. In sharing the meal together, we *become* the body and blood of Christ.

Because these ordinary items are key parts of how we tell and live into the story of Jesus, we cannot simply toss the leftovers into the garbage. Instead, we honor the purpose for which we offered them. The word "ablutions" refers to our careful actions with the leftover bread and wine. It is right that they be consumed in the same manner of prayer, thanksgiving, reflection, hope, community, and relationship in which we consumed them during worship. If there is too much bread and wine left over, it can be carefully disposed of in the ways that are typically considered respectful to a corpse: consumed by flame or buried in the ground.

Our care and attention to the crumbs of bread and the dregs of wine are an invitation to be more attentive and grateful for all of the gifts God gives us, for all of the parts of God's creation that give us life. It is the antithesis of the wastefulness that is the norm in our disposable society.

The Living Diet

Thanksgiving

We come now to the first part of the Living Diet. Out of our personal and faith stories, patterns emerge, possibilities for living. I want to state clearly that this diet is not to be received as a list of rules, but rather as a gentle framework that individuals, families, and communities, in a variety of circumstances and configurations, can adopt by choosing the parts that best speak to you. May you find these simple practices liberating. May they offer a new form to your life that allows you to reclaim your real nature: your body inextricably connected to mind and spirit, inextricably connected to the world around you. In becoming more real, may you find health and joy.

Grace

The blessing of food is a raucous affair in our home. Our children have a table prayer that they sing to the tune of "Doo Wah Diddy Diddy."

"*Thank you Lord for the food that we receive, singing doo wah diddy diddy,*" it begins. In biblical accounts, whenever Jesus shared a meal he was said to "bless and break" the food first. When he did so, the food became a means of recognition. The food was recognized as blessing and the meal was recognized as a sign of God's barrier-breaking love. People were recognized as fed, welcomed, and healed. Jesus was recognized as the human face of God's love, present to all on the journey.

The act of giving thanks for our food before we eat is a consistent way of recognizing that food is not merely about us. It is a means to reconfigure our mindless eating and ask for our eyes to be opened to the blessings we have, as well as the blessings that are possible as we ourselves bless, break, and share.

The cloudy-vs-crystalline images of the water molecule experiment discussed at the beginning of this chapter remind us that reconfiguration takes place both in the cells that make up the food that we eat, as well as in the cells that constitute the bodies that we are feeding. In other words, the physical world in which we are given life, sustained in life, connected in life, is changed by our choice to eat with thought, care, attentiveness, and gratitude.

A prayer of thanksgiving over our food is a concrete first step in the Living Diet. You may have young children who love to lead in a fun and feisty prayer, or you might feel comfortable ad-libbing words of gratitude. My mother owns a book of seasonally appropriate table blessings that provides prayers of simple beauty but takes the pressure off having to come up with the right words herself. Some people take a moment of silent thanks before beginning to eat. It can be particularly meaningful to offer a brief prayer of thanksgiving when dining out. A pause, a head bowed, a single moment of praise and blessing is so rarely seen in public space that it can both ground the person offering the prayer, as well as stand in quiet witness to others of a different attitude toward the gifts we receive at table. Although I was brought up in this secular culture to feel an almost allergic reaction to "pushing" my religion on anyone, I find that nonreligious guests around my own family's table are nonetheless respectful of our family's tradition of table blessing and join in the thanksgiving without qualm.

Thanksgiving for Meat

We were in Nova Scotia with my parents and my brother's family for Mom and Dad's fortieth wedding anniversary. It seemed fitting to mark this special occasion with a seafood feast. Dan and my dad were tasked with sourcing the lobster, while my brother, sister-in-law, and I went into town to buy the accompaniments. When we all arrived back at our rented cottage, there were seven live lobsters puttering around an enormous storage bin on the patio. They elicited worried conversation throughout the day. Were they okay in that bin? They looked miserable, but then lobsters have a sort of grim appearance at the best of times. More importantly, who was going to kill them, and how?

"You need two people," someone in the group offered. "One to hold the lobster over the boiling water while the other person clips the elastic band off their claws."

I was grateful when Dan volunteered to take charge of the operation. He was worried about the deed, but he put his worry to good use, researching the best and most ethical way to kill the animals that would become our dinner. He learned that boiling them alive had been proven to be inhumane and torturous, but that a quick severing of their neck prior to cooking was considered painless.

Our children, ages six and eight at the time, found themselves consumed with worry and care for the lobsters. We have always talked openly about the fact that meat comes from animals. Cecilia loves seafood and was looking forward to eating lobster at the feast. She wasn't worried about eating an animal that had been alive that day, but she was prompted by the whole experience to join her dad in saying a prayer before he slaughtered the animals. She and Gordon included the lobsters in both the grace that they led at supper and in their night prayers.

We eat meat more regularly than I would like in our household. Yet, in this one act we were faced with the fact that our meat was provided to us by real creatures. We were literally holding their lives in our hands, and we had both a responsibility and a gift by being entrusted with killing, cooking, and consuming them. Our experience brought home the physicality of eating meat in a way that yielded care and gratitude.

There are Christian reasons for refraining from eating meat. I will talk about some of them in a later chapter. For those who do eat meat, the reality is that a sacrifice of life takes place that we might draw nourishment from the food. In hunting, fishing, or farming societies, the connection between human and animal is undeniable and viscerally experienced. The family eating the meat knows firsthand the experience of raising, feeding, nurturing, slaughtering, hunting, and then preparing the animal they will eat. A childhood book I loved, *Little House in the Big Woods*, goes into lengthy detail describing a wild pig hunted and brought home by Laura's "Pa"—how the pig was prepared and used, and how every piece of the animal provided sustenance and joy for the family consuming it, right down to the tail (the crispy treat shared by the children) and the bladder (blown up and played with as a toy balloon).

Benedict, in his Rule of Life, called the Brothers to fast from the "flesh of four-footed animals," although this rule could be lifted for "the very weak and sick."[3] Fr. Charles Cummings, a Trappist monk, takes a lighter stance on the issue. He advocates for the flexibility of choice in meat-eating, but insists that, whatever the choice, it be grounded in gratitude: "Those who eat, eat in honor of the Lord, since they give thanks to God; while those who abstain, abstain in honor of the Lord and give thanks to God" (1 Cor. 8:13; Rom 14:20).[4] Although we have lost much of the personal relationship with the animals we eat, something of that blessing can be restored by offering a specific prayer of thanksgiving when meat is part of our meal.

Become a Caretaker of the Water

In First Nations' communities, women are traditionally responsible for the care of the water. As the Sisterhood of the Planetary Water Rites group notes:

---

3. *The Rule of Saint Benedict*, ed. J. Connor Gallagher (Charlotte, NC: Saint Benedict Press, 2007), chapter 39, verse 11, page 66.

4. Mary Margaret Funk, *Thoughts Matter: Discovering the Spiritual Journey* (New York: Continuum, 1998), 27.

We have the connection and the ways and the ceremonies to bless and purify our waters as well as the waters that make up 70% of our physical bodies.

We are living in the days of the great purification of the Earth. We have the choice to sit by helplessly watching the events take place or to be active participants in easing her passage. It can be as simple as singing a song at a river bank, putting our hands over a bowl of water for our children's consumption, giving thanks and blessing the water that goes into our morning coffee, or picking up the garbage at the beach.[5]

Jesus, in a similar vein, identified himself as the one who gives living water—those who come to him will never be thirsty (John 4:13) and out of the heart of those who believe in him will flow living waters (John 7:38).

Given that all life consists primarily of water, given the ability to physically impact that water through the words we choose to say over it, and given the devastation caused by our misuse of this most basic staple of life as a cheap and disposable resource, perhaps we should all take on the role of keepers of the water. We can embrace the First Nations' wisdom around water. Rather than merely worship Jesus as the Water of Life, we can follow where this Living Water leads: baptized through the water, to become the life that springs forth for the sake of others.

That may sound a strange and esoteric order. But being a keeper of the water, embracing our Christ-like role, begins with simple steps that change the way we care for ourselves and the world around us; simple steps that change our bodies that are both sustained and killed by water—clean or polluted, blessed or ignored, nurtured or abused.

- Make a daily habit of giving thanks for the blessing of water: hot water in which to bathe; cool water in which to be refreshed; clean water to drink; lakes and streams and rivers and oceans of water that connect and nourish our world, steal our breath with their beauty.

---

5. From the introduction to the "Nibi Wabo Water Ceremony" by The Sisterhood of the Planetary Water Rites, *http://www.waterblessings.org/ceremonies_general.html*.

- As you pray with gratitude, pray also with compassion. Pray for clean water to be made available to all of our siblings around the world.
- Look for opportunities to address the water needs—through charitable giving, advocacy, education, and partnership—of communities in our world and our nation that do not have access to clean water.
- Notice how our commitment to the water needs of others changes the way in which we see and consume water in our own daily lives.

Ablutions

Earlier I spoke about the ablutions that follow the eucharistic meal we share in church. It is an act of taking care with what has been blessed to our use. Because we understand the bread and the wine as revealing to us the body and blood of Christ, we are responsible for honoring that bread and wine accordingly.

The act of ablutions can also be carried into our kitchens and dining rooms. By no means does this have to become oppressive or inflexible, but we can defy the norm of wastefulness—that all-too-common picture of the half-eaten restaurant meal with a napkin crumpled on top to signal to the server that it is finished. Imagine if we treated the food and drink from our tables with the same care we treat the bread and wine at communion. We would bring our own take-out container to restaurants so that extra food could be brought home. We would save leftovers and plan how to put them to future use. We would carefully scrape plates and sort the scraps into our green bins or compost piles, returning them to the earth to continue in the purpose for which God created them. Because our eyes see water as precious and life-giving, we would take only what we intend to drink. When we host parties or get-togethers, we would insist that a green bin be available in a central location so that those half-eaten pieces of cake and their paper napkin companions might be properly disposed of.

Our thoughtfulness can extend to before the meal as well. My grandmother, with Depression-era frugality, taught me well in the art of the strong spatula. If I was baking in her kitchen, my bowls had to be thoroughly scraped down, every lick of my concoction swept into the finished product going into the oven. Of course, this deeply disappointed me as a child. I think that I only baked in order to scrape out and eat the leftover batter! If you have kids at home, you might opt for a weaker spatula and let licking the bowl clean be part of the ablutions.

Part of this practice is choosing our portions more carefully. All-you-can-eat Japanese restaurants have been springing up in our city lately. In contrast to the all-you-can-eat Chinese buffets with which many of us are familiar, these new places make the food fresh-to-order. There is one caveat: you can order as much as you want, *but you have to eat it.* Some will even go as far as to charge you extra for the dishes you order and don't consume. We, likewise, can learn to pick our portions with an orientation toward the simple rule of planning to eat what we take.

Daily Examen

Ultimately Eucharist doesn't refer to some act in which Jesus engaged. It doesn't refer to an hour-plus we might spend in a church building in a week. It doesn't even just extend into a particular attitude toward our food. Eucharist is a way of life in which our eyes are continually opening in recognition and then gratitude for the blessings around us. It is a way of life that could be compared to that of an athlete in training: we engage in a daily regimen of exercise to develop our muscles of gratitude.

One of the simple ways of deepening this training and increasing our capacity for this gratitude is an ancient practice called the Daily Examen. As the day is drawing to a close, we pause for a few moments. We review what has happened since we got out of bed that morning: for what are we grateful, for whom are we grateful, what challenges did we experience, and what grace were we given to meet them? The Daily Examen naturally leads to questions of regret and disappointment. Where do we feel a sense of failure in our choices? Our honesty becomes a part of our gratitude training. When we can name our faults, we can seek forgiveness and renewal. We can make the connection between what we have received and what we have done. We can develop our capacity for making that connection stronger and more visible—the thanks we give leads us to a life that can be more generous and other-centered.

Daily practices of gratitude may seem unrelated to food and body issues. I would argue instead that *they are the missing piece* in even the best dieting advice columns and self-help books. Without practices of gratitude, we concentrate only on the food we choose to eat and the bodies we have as a result, with no reference to how our food and our bodies live and move in the world. We ignore how our food and our bodies can *serve* the world. Instead, we buy into the reductionist food/body worldview that imprisons so many of us. In contrast, our words of gratitude for our food lead us into actions of care for God's gifts, strengthen our muscles of recognition and thanksgiving, and loop us back into an increased awareness of the blessing of food.

Giving It Away

There is a final step in this feedback loop of gratitude. I need to learn to give away. Our churches teach us to consider our financial gifts. Before I use any of my money for my family or myself, I choose to give a portion of it away. In biblical language, this off-the-top giving is called the firstfruits. When I give in this planned and proportionate way, I notice how my attitude toward my resources is transformed, how I become aware of abundance. I discover that I can give first, and I still have more than what I need. Gratitude and generosity feed off one another, each muscle group strengthening the other when exercised regularly.

You can give to your faith community, or you can give to a charity with which you feel most aligned. If you yourself do not belong to a community of faith, you can choose one that best reflects your values in their work in the world and their care of one another and give to them. And you can choose how much. The power is in the choice and planning, not in the amount. Start with 1 or 2 percent of your income or start with giving away one hour's wage a week. As you notice the impact of this practice—particularly as you start to notice how much you still have—you might then choose to increase what you give away.

I Don't Know I'm Hungry

once gave up sugar, wheat, corn, dairy, caffeine, and alcohol for a period of two months. There were complex reasons behind what I considered to be a truly heroic stint of abstinence. I had been feeling increasingly worn out and was regularly short with the people closest to me. I was also training for a half marathon. I decided to see Gloria, a parishioner of mine who was a registered nurse and operated a nutrition counseling business from her home. She was known around town as a healer and wonder worker. She had recommended the diet in order to "take stress off my system." Her theory was that these foods cause inflammation, which could account for the fatigue, stress, and moodiness I had been experiencing.

I was excited about the "new me" she promised in her eating advice. Although I would never have said so out loud, I also immediately began to imagine that this "new me" would be thinner. I hadn't dieted, hadn't even weighed myself, in the ten years since my strange vision of Jesus's healing. Yet I was too well indoctrinated by the weight loss culture around me to not associate such a radical change in eating with a shrinking waistline. I could almost hear the comments, the same ones that I had so longed to hear a decade before: "Wow, you look great! Have you lost weight?"

I followed her advice stoically. I promptly experienced a debilitating drop in energy. If I had been moody before, it was nothing compared to the snappish irritability that emerged two weeks in to my new routine, culminating with my picking a fight with my brother over some trivial slight and then weeping inconsolably in front of my family until they insisted that I go back to Gloria and tell her that this eating regimen was clearly not working.

Gloria was as baffled by my bad reaction to clean eating as I was, so she took me to see a friend of hers, a trainer in town who was a competitive weight lifter. The gym was in the basement of a strip mall. I could tell immediately that this was a different class of athlete than I was used to seeing at the local YMCA. Nobody looked like they had just rolled off the couch to begin breaking entrenched habits of inactivity. These were people of experience. I recognized the room as the one that I used to visit with my mom. It had previously been a fabric store, and I would wait, struggling to be patient, for the several eternities it took Mom to happily pore over the patterns and colors and sales. The short, muscular man to whom Gloria introduced me looked like Bernie, the hotel manager from the movie *Pretty Woman*. Gloria outlined my problem and my goal. "She's running a half marathon in a couple of weeks."

"Okay, tell me what you're eating," he said briskly. I described, with some defensiveness and a touch of pride, my new regime of quinoa, lentils, and other whole and natural foods, along with all of the salad, veggies, and fruit I was already used to.

"You can't run a half marathon," he said with an air of finality. "You're starving yourself." I responded with shocked silence, so he elaborated, "You can't do what you're doing and not eat enough."

"Not enough?" I murmured.

"You're starving yourself," he repeated. "Where is the complex protein? Where are the snacks? You need to be eating protein to repair and build muscles. You need to get serious about carbs. No wonder you're falling apart. You have burned out your body. And you're going to do serious damage if you continue."

I racked my muddled and discouraged brain for all of the reasons why that couldn't be right. "B-b-b-ut," I stumbled out, "I haven't lost any weight. I can't possibly be not eating enough. My weight hasn't budged."

"And it won't," he countered. "The body will hoard fat and burn muscle if it's not being properly fed. You have to eat enough to lose weight."

If the floor of the gym had split open at that moment and swallowed me whole, I would have been less thunderstruck than I was by his statement. After outlining a regimen of complex proteins and carbs at all three meals, with energy-rich snacks in between, he softened. "How long until your half marathon?" I told him that I was two weeks out. "If you want to do it just to do it, if you eat really well and carefully between now and then, if you don't push yourself to an extreme when you're racing, you can do it. You can try it. Otherwise you could do damage that could take six months to recover from."

On the drive back, I expressed my doubts to Gloria by falling back on that one equation we all understand: "I didn't do any of this to lose weight," I said out loud once again, also to convince myself. "But I don't want to *gain* weight either," I finished in a small voice. Eating more? My daydreams shifted away from my earlier excitement of eating better and looking better, and instead spiraled right into the iron grip of the fear of getting fat. Eat proteins and carbs first, Bernie had told me, only if you have room after can you eat veggies and fruit. What kind of advice was that?

"You won't gain weight," Gloria promised me. "Fat doesn't come from eating too much. It's protection. It's the body protecting itself." Her response vaguely registered in my mind as consistent with her theory of inflammation—the body protecting itself.

But it was hard to hear her for all of the competing voices and memories crowding my mind. What about the reductionist understanding of the equation between food and our bodies in all those women's magazine articles that said if I consumed a hundred extra calories a day, I would put on an extra ten pounds a year? What about those celebrity diets that say the route to a perfect body is through tightly controlled portion sizes of approved types of food along with punishing regimes of physical exercise? What about my first-year university roommate Ty, a kinesiology student and varsity athlete who would count out seventeen Doritos because she had calculated the exact number of calories she could safely consume without adding extra fat to her perfect body? What about her constant advice that if I wanted to lose weight I just needed to decrease my calories and increase my physical exercise? What about Weight Watchers? Calorie Counters? Online apps for tracking calories and points?

I had been talking for ten years about learning to love and respect our bodies, to love and enjoy our relationship with food. And here, in the space of a half hour, I was locked in a showdown with all of the hang-ups I still carried around. The Doritos and the Weight Watchers and the celebrity diets were the foundation on which I had unknowingly continued to build my relationship between food and my body.

I believed that being hungry at the end of the day was good. I believed that eating less was always better, nobler, and led to desirable results. Deep down inside, underneath the healing and the freedom I had experienced, *I still feared my own body.* I did not trust it to communicate its hunger and its need. I did not know how to listen to it and to feed myself. I still saw overeating as a shame to be hidden, not ever imagining that so-called overeating could be redefined as healthy and good. I feared an out-of-control appetite and an irrepressibly expanding midsection.

"Is eating this complicated for everyone, or just you?" a friend asked in a concerned voice. It was a telling comment. We see regular eating of good food as complicated. I began the diet because I was feeling worn out. And yet, my worn-out life was bringing me back to this one basic relationship. Did I understand hunger? Did I respect and trust my body enough to listen to that hunger and feed it?

An Honest Hungry

> Charity had always slightly creeped me out: There was nothing quite as condescending as the phrase "helping the less fortunate" rolling off the tongue of a white professional, as if poverty were a matter of luck instead of the result of a political system. . . . And yet . . . there was that vision of a Table where everyone was welcome. Our neighbors, friends and strangers, were hungry. The very least a Christian church could do, for starters, was feed them.
>
> —Sara Miles, *Take This Bread*[1]

About the same time that I was trying to sift my way through the mysteries of wheat-free bread recipes and boiling down fruit to make icing without refined sugar, a young man showed up for St. David's worship

1. Sara Miles, *Take This Bread: A Radical Conversion* (New York: Random House, 2007), 107–8.

service one Sunday morning. With little prompting, he began to share his story with me. He had grown up in a family in which drug and physical abuse ran rampant. Diagnosed as bipolar at a young age, he was on a series of complicated medications and the previous year had instigated an armed robbery, an incident he claimed was fueled by a bad reaction between alcohol and medication. He had just gotten out of jail and was living in a rooming house, trying to piece his life back together, to find employment, to be a good father to his two daughters, and to feel his way forward out of the family patterns that he had so easily fallen into repeating.

He worshipped with us. When the table had been prepared, the wine poured, the bread blessed and broken, I issued the invitation we always issue: "This is the table at which God is host and all are welcome guests."[2] Before the choir, servers, and worship assistants could gather around the altar to receive communion, Dennis walked up from the back of the church, past the communion railing, up the three steps separating the sanctuary from the rest of the church, stood in front of me and put his hands out ready to receive.

I gave him the bread. The communion assistant gave him the wine. He was visibly moved by the experience and worshipped with us over the course of the few months in which his life was stable enough that he lived within walking distance of the church.

Dennis received something that morning. But to an even more significant degree, our congregation received something. He startled us. So often we find ourselves going to church half asleep and coming up to communion simply doing that thing that we always do. It was a surprise to see his eagerness transcend the protocol and reserve we normally associate with mainline religious practice. Dennis couldn't wait. He reminded us of what it means to want—to desperately, physically, spiritually, mentally, and emotionally hunger for what God has to offer.

No doubt God had a hand in leading Dennis to us that morning. But there were also practical circumstances that opened the door to him. St. David's offers a free meal on Sunday morning. He came

---

2. My friend and supervisor Michael, with whom I worked in my first parish, had crafted this wording. "I think it's important for people to hear explicitly *who* is doing the inviting," he would say.

to church because he was hungry. The church had begun a community breakfast program a few years earlier. They decided to offer the breakfast on Sunday mornings for a few important reasons. For one thing, there were no feeding programs being offered on the weekends in Orillia. But more importantly, Sunday was when the church was assembled, when they had the best possibility of making the meal about more than filling bellies once a week. Members of the church were encouraged to share in the breakfast too. It became an offering of food in response to real physical hunger, but they were also offering and receiving community. People were asked to invest in eating, speaking to, and coming to know one another, whether they had money or not, whether they were physically hungry or not, whether they attended church or not.

St. David's is a small congregation. When the community breakfast was first proposed, the church felt anxiety and hesitation about taking on such a big commitment. Within months, however, the breakfast had become an integral part of their identity. A wide variety of people continue to come through the doors every Sunday: single mothers, temporarily unemployed, continually unemployed, underemployed, families living in affordable housing units, families who wait to live in affordable housing units, seniors, addicts. There are people who regularly ask for hand-outs, responding to whatever is given with, "Could you give more?" And there are people who might be too proud to accept a free meal, but who are able to look around and see everyone enjoying the food, and in that community feel able to receive something they need too. The conversation around the tables is diverse and unruly, everything from politics to the weather to religion, from the banal to the serious. As the clock drifts closer to the 10 a.m. worship time, the guests continue on into their days, or linger a little longer over breakfast, or come upstairs for worship. There is no pressure to do so, but many have found their way in to share in the community's prayer and praise.

While I have now moved on to leadership in another parish, St. David's continues its breakfast program. They are addressing a need. They are becoming a welcoming, safe, and vital space within their neighborhood. They have an ongoing connection with the people who

live closest to the church building. But the breakfast has been meaningful and transformative in another way. St. David's has found itself, not
just on the offering end of a transaction, but also on the receiving end.

When You Offer Food, You Don't Get to Decide Who Will Show Up

We should expect that when we feed others, we ourselves will be
changed. When we offer food, hungry people turn up. When Jesus
enacted a realm where all people were fed and valued, the implications
challenged him as well. A Syrophoenician woman asked that he look
beyond his own preconceived ideas of who mattered, for whom his
ministry was offered (Mark 7:24–30). A foolish courage led Jesus into
the land of the Gerasenes and a frightening graveyard encounter with
a man isolated by every category imaginable: race, circumstance, and
location (Mark 5:1–20). Each of the gospel accounts bears witness to a
ministry that evolved to include women in subversive new ways, to the
point that a nameless woman outsider became God's priest, anointing
Jesus before his death (Mark 14:3–9).

When we offer food, hungry people turn up and we must relinquish
control. The hunger that Jesus encountered in his ministry changed how
he viewed the world, how he understood God, and how he enacted his
ministry. His encounters with the spiritual and physical hunger of those
he met created a feedback loop that expanded the gospel to include
people Jesus initially assumed had nothing to do with him. As the gospel expanded, Jesus became more outspoken about and compassionate
toward the needs of those around him. As he became more outspoken,
his ministry became more precarious and the forces of darkness con-
spired to silence him. As his life narrowed toward its violent end, Jesus
was able to lift up food and table fellowship as the vehicle through which
his life and ministry would continue. In the Resurrection, broken bread
is forever transformed for those who are bound to Jesus.

Likewise, at St. David's, as the church gathers for the main worship
of the community, the boundaries between who belongs and who doesn't
break down, even as the doors of the church building open up. Food is
offered, and in doing so, control is surrendered, because when we offer

to feed people, we do not get to decide which of the hungry will show up. As Carmelite John Welch says, "The hunger within us is so deep and powerful that, acknowledged or not, only God is sufficient food."[3] The obvious need of the people who come to church because there is food reminds us that need isn't what divides the "us" from the "them." Need is what unites us. Whether on a conscious level or not, the Eucharist leads us into the act of coming forward, hands outstretched to physically acknowledge that we cannot go it alone, that there is an empty place in each of us that can only be filled by God. Welch continues:

> We humans never have enough because we choose All. And we never rest until we get it. We are made this way. Made to seek and search, yearn and ache, until the heart finally finds something or someone to match the depth of its desire, until the heart finds food sufficient for its hunger.[4]

Are You Hungry?

Controversial table fellowship weaves through the accounts of Jesus's ministry, and the gospels establish that hunger, in all of its various manifestations, is the starting point for discipleship. Early on, Jesus encountered resistance from some of the religious leaders. He responded with this simple parable: "Those who are well have no need of a physician, but those who are sick" (Luke 5:31). Jesus asked his curious listeners to look inside themselves and identify whether or not they *needed*. Former Archbishop of Canterbury Rowan Williams commented on the text:

> "If you don't think you need me," Jesus says to the strict believers, "feel free to go." And we might think he looks each one of them in the eye and says, "So, do you need me or not? Are you hungry? Are you sick? Is your work, your life unfinished? Because, if you are whole and not hungry, and finished, go."[5]

---

3. John Welch, *Seasons of the Heart* (Darien, IL: Carmelite Communications Center, 2008), 4.

4. Ibid.

5. Sermon given Sunday, June 26, 2005, at the Diocesan Celebration for the 13th Meeting of the Anglican Consultative Council, Nottingham, England.

Williams hits on a pattern of discipleship that consistently marks the moments of world-changing redirection in the story of our faith: tasting then seeing; the surprising, sweet, unmerited bread of life offered and received into our stomachs before our eyes are opened to see the God who has been there all along. He defines the church in this way:

> Here we are, then, the people who have not found the nerve to walk away. And is that perhaps the best definition we could have of the Church? We are the people who have not had the nerve to walk away; who have not had the nerve to say in the face of Jesus, "All right, I'm healthy, I'm not hungry. I'm finished, I'm done." We're here as hungry people, we are here because we cannot heal and complete ourselves; we're here to eat together at the table of the Lord, as he sits at dinner in this house, and is surrounded by these disreputable, unfinished, unhealthy, hungry, sinful, but at the end of the day almost honest people, gathered with him to find renewal, to be converted, and to change.[6]

As we are invited to follow in Jesus's way, we, too, learn to identify hunger and to discern how God might be using us to feed the hunger in others. But this ministry is never one way. When we learn something about our world's hunger and how God might be addressing it, we also learn something about ourselves.

Do you remember my story of nursing my insatiable infant daughter Cecilia? The learning I eventually received was this: *we are born hungry.* The act of eating is ultimately an opportunity to be honest. We do not go it alone. Each of us is biologically configured to require life from outside of ourselves in order to live.

God's Table, Our Tables

The ways in which Jesus was transformed by his recognition of hunger, and his actions of hospitality in the face of that hunger, translate into twenty-first-century Christians' relationship with food. How we eat and what we eat matters to God; it matters very much.

---

6. Ibid.

The next step in St. David's ministry of feeding was to expand both the community breakfast and the worship practices to make the connection between God's table, the community table, and our home tables. Without prompting, people simply started bringing food to worship for those who were a little closer to the edge of desperation.

I watched this impulse evolve at St. David's, but it is hardly unique. Many congregations take gifts of food up to the altar at the same time as they are taking forward gifts of money and the bread and wine to be shared at God's table. In Sara Miles's book *Take This Bread*, she describes her own radical conversion to Christianity and the resulting initiative to gather food donations from various community sources onto the altar in the center of her church's worship space, and to invite those who were hungry to take the food.

Many of our parishioners at my current church of St. George have long been in the habit of bringing nonperishable food with them each week for the Community Care barrels at the back of the church. And most able-bodied members of the congregation volunteer at least once a month on one of the thirty-one breakfast teams that are each responsible for providing a free hot breakfast to anyone who shows up, 365 days of the year. We recently began a monthly community dinner, which again is meant to be something other than an offering of charity, but rather an experience of how people of diverse means and circumstances are bound together by the common need to eat and the common joy of eating together.

In bringing our gifts to God's table and then extending those gifts out to meet the world's need, we demonstrate the truth that we can't be honest about our own hunger without also experiencing compassion for the hunger of others. We have misunderstood the hunger of others if we don't also recognize our own emptiness, need, and brokenness—our own hunger.

Hunger: An Antidote to Isolation

Our unhealthy twenty-first-century relationship with food isn't actually about the chemicals, preservatives, and hormones we pump into our meat and onto our produce; it isn't about eating too much; it isn't about eating the wrong things; it isn't about sugar and trans fats, sugar substitutes, or brown rice. The poor quality of health in our Western eating habits is fundamentally grounded in the lie that our bodies are disconnected from the world around us. Our disconnected bodies then become autonomous organisms ripe for indulgence and trickery. We cave to the persuasion of the multi-trillion-dollar advertising, junk food, diet food, and health food industries. We buy into the persistent assumption that we are at war with our bodies. We are cut off from the relationship that actually feeds us. We learn to deny the connection between body and soul—between bodies and souls.

Hunger is the reconnector. Theologian Richard Rohr reflects on the worship of the church and Eucharist with these words:

> The Eucharist is telling us that God is the food and all we have to do is provide the hunger. Somehow we have to make sure that each day we are hungry, that there's room inside of us for another presence. If you are filled with your own opinions, ideas, righteousness, superiority, or sufficiency, you are a world unto yourself and there is no room for "another."[7]

His words are applicable well outside the confines of worship. Each day, we need to be honest about our physical hunger so that we can be intentional about seeking the things that will feed our deeper hunger. Then we can be more mindful about not filling our souls and bodies with junk. Each day, we need to learn to be compassionate toward the needs of others, not because we pity them, but because we understand something of our own vulnerability and how it connects us. Then we can be more attentive to creating a world where there is good food for all. Each day, I can be reacquainted with my own hunger and that of my siblings. I can also turn my eating away from distrust, indulgence, and guilt, and toward my God-given capacity for gratitude and generosity, both of which are postures fundamentally necessary for health and wellness.

---

7. Richard Rohr, "Make Sure You Are Hungry," Richard Rohr's Daily Meditations (13 out of 53), *The Centre for Action and Contemplation*, August 8. 2013, *https://myemail.constantcontact.com/Richard-Rohr-s-Daily-Meditations--Make-Sure-You-Are-Hungry----Transformation----August-8--2013.html?soid=1103098668616&aid=RKQqaj_20TE.*

The Living Diet

Hungering

If I am full—self-made, independent, satisfied, and complete—I am isolated. I am cut off from the truth of who I am: the truth built into the act of eating. I lose my identity as a relationship and become merely a consumer, manipulated into buying-ingesting-voiding consumables. I am left simultaneously bloated and empty.

Alternatively, if I understand myself as hungry—as needing something or someone beyond myself—I am equipped to repel so many of the destructive food messages constantly being launched at me. What follows is a series of possibilities for reconnecting with our hunger.

Shopping Weekly for the Food Bank

When you are grocery shopping for your own household tables, pick up a few, or even just one extra item of nonperishable food to give to a food bank. Many grocery stores now provide bins so you can make your donation on the spot. As you are trying to make your own thoughtful and conscientious choices for the food you will eat, allow the regular consideration of the hunger of others and the need in your community to be part of your purchasing practice.

Participating in a Feeding Program

For my first-year field placement at seminary, the internship director suggested that I volunteer at a soup kitchen in the Regent Park area of Toronto. I wasn't familiar with the various neighborhoods of the city nor the reputation of each, but when I met with my supervisor (a Salvation Army captain), she explained that Regent Park was one of the most challenged parts of the city. "All kinds of social resources are being pumped into this area all the time," she told me. "But we don't necessarily see the money doing a lot of good in breaking cycles." She went on to tell me that her expectation of me at the soup kitchen wasn't that I would make food. "What we find makes a difference in people's lives, in helping to break cycles of poverty and addiction, is relationship. You're not here to make food. You're here to get to know people." I subsequently went in each Friday morning. As promised, the culinary expectations were minimal. We served hot coffee and leftover donated doughnuts and muffins. I was in the kitchen to assemble the supplies and turn the coffee on. Then I spent the morning drinking coffee with the guests.

I was intimidated at first. I was suddenly aware of the privilege I had enjoyed, and taken for granted, all of my life. My parents not only made sure that I was fed and clothed and educated, they also made it possible for me to take a variety of music lessons and go on band trips. I worried about what kind of clothes I would wear, not whether I would have clothes. I fretted about offending my parents by not liking the food they had made. I never wondered if there would be food on the table. I went to bed at night hoping that I had aced my math test, all the while assuming that a world of opportunity lay before me. I dabbled in alcohol and tried to make decisions around friends and social occasions with some integrity and sense of responsibility; substance abuse was not an escape from the cultural and economic patterns that left me feeling hopeless. I had no experience with the kind of need that this group knew and lived.

It didn't matter. We talked about our families and the weather. We talked politics and religion and current events. They told me amazing stories of conversion and faith. We told jokes. I prayed for them and they prayed for me. Sometimes we just sat in companionable silence drinking our coffee. I needn't have worried about the divide that I assumed would be between us. Common ground is surprisingly easy to find, even between people who seem to have come from totally different backgrounds and who are living in entirely different circumstances. We all cared about being close to our loved ones and making meaning of the world around us.

Becoming a volunteer at a soup kitchen, a weekend feeding program, or a food bank will change your familiarity with hunger in your community and in yourself. If you think you don't have time, try attending one of these meals on a periodic basis. If you are concerned about eating the food that is meant for people without financial means, you can make a contribution to the program in return. Whether you are a volunteer or a participant, take time to talk with others who attend the program. Discover the connections between your life and theirs. Be attentive to the differences; listen and learn from their experiences. When we break bread together, we learn we are no longer strangers living in separate worlds.

Praying and Meditating

In time set aside for prayer, meditation, contemplation, or simple quiet, reflect on your own questions of hunger: What do I desire? Where and to what am I being drawn? Allow your reflection to clarify the difference between what you want and what you need. Give thanks for how your needs have been met. Ask for generosity in sharing your own abundance with others. Surrender the need, the longing, the desire, and the hunger that you experience in your own life. Turn over that emptiness to a power—a love—that is big enough to hold and fill you. And when you still feel empty, or you feel empty again, surrender one more time. And one more time. Make a daily practice of offering up your hunger.

Remembering the Story

In the Hebrew Scriptures, the people of Israel entered into the Promised Land and were immediately told to sit down and share a meal. What's more, they were tasked with sitting down regularly to share in the feasts of their faith, particularly the annual celebration of Passover. Along with the meal came the observance of first fruits—a practice of offering back to God a portion of everything each household has received that season. As the offering was made they recounted their people's story of slavery in Egypt and of deliverance and provision through God's "mighty hand" (Deut. 26:5–10).

Jesus's people were to receive with joy all of the blessings of harvest, food, the fellowship and celebration that goes along with the observance of the feast. In the midst of that, they kept track of their own ancestral story of hunger, and within that story the remembrance of grace and blessing.

There is no family or religious history that does not include stories of need and experiences of provision. Taking time to share these stories and to reflect on them changes our attitude toward food. Food moves from being a commodity to be consumed to being a gift we receive and use toward a purpose larger than our own fulfillment. As the passage ends, "When you have finished paying all the tithe of your produce in the third year (which is the year of the tithe), giving it to the Levites, the aliens, the orphans, and the widows, so that they may eat their fill within your towns" (Deut. 26:12).

Food Is Personal

My friend Erin went vegan and lost seventeen pounds. She described her new diet and the reasons behind it to our group of girlfriends at a summer get-together. It was as simple, she told us, as getting her hands on the right health and weight-loss research. "My body just can't process animal fat," she explained. "If I try those low carb, high protein diets, I just put on weight."

It doesn't seem to matter how evolved we are, how firmly we have come to define ourselves as succeeding in the battle of accepting our bodies (and therefore ourselves), we can't seem to help but be drawn in by a witness who claims they have found the secret to effortless weight loss. Another friend, Alex, interrogated Erin about the ins and outs of this radical lifestyle change.

"Well," Alex concluded, "good for you." And then, as if she were stating the obvious, "I mean, veganism is crazy. If you were doing it to like *save the environment*, or something ridiculous like that, I would definitely *not* be supportive. But for personal reasons, health, trimming up, I think that's great."

We had had a day of swimming, watching our kids play together, joking and giggling about the blisses and challenges of our careers, families, and parenting, in the effortless way that good friendship affords. But it was Alex's words that rattled in my head at the end of the day. Given our current global reality, with every summer breaking the heat records of the previous summer, with countless numbers of people dying in California wildfires one year and Pakistan's deadly floods another, not to mention the devastation of climate change hitting closer and closer to home, how could any thoughtful person not care about trying to make lifestyle changes to alleviate some of the pressure on our fragile climate? And, more than that, how could they be blatantly condemning of any attempts others make toward that necessary change? Despite the overwhelming nature of the climate change story (*what can one person really do?*), the truth remains that our individual choices matter.

In fact, what we eat is perhaps the most important decision we make in how we want our world to be structured. It is our daily vote about what kind of future we want. Producing one calorie from animal protein requires eleven times as much fossil fuel, releasing eleven times as much carbon dioxide, as producing one calorie from plant protein. Studies estimate that a vegan is responsible for seven times *less* carbon dioxide emissions than a meat-eater. Not only does the raising, slaughtering, and transporting of animals produce carbon dioxide, it also produces excessive quantities of methane, a gas thought to be twenty times more effective than CO_2 at trapping heat in our atmosphere.

I was caught off guard by Alex and didn't manage to climb up on my soapbox to fight for the dignity of our planet and the need for conscientious, global-oriented decision making. I didn't point out the destructive selfishness of an attitude that is killing our world and therefore killing us. And given that I value our friendship, and that I was eating a hamburger at the time, it's certainly best that I didn't.

"The only reason I *would* consider being vegan is for environmental reasons," I muttered into my sandwich. After all, my current non-veggie status didn't allow me to throw stones at other people's carnivore houses. The conversation politely moved on to other things.

Our planet is in crisis, and we are immobilized, unable, or unwilling to make a move. It's not just Alex who doesn't care. Politicians are being elected across North America on climate change *denying* platforms, or platforms that insist that carbon taxes should be eliminated, or that emission-reducing targets need not be considered important. Human responsibility in the reality of global warming continues to be questioned, which all of the evidence suggests is a victory for the PR machine more than an actual conflict in the research. But it seems to me that the greatest reason for our unwillingness to fight this issue is not that seeds of doubt have managed to be sown by the privately funded research of oil companies, although that doesn't help. Instead, I think that the crux of it can be found in a closer examination of Alex's words.

It's not personal. Climate change is not personal. Alex gave me some insight into her resistance when she followed up her strident response to meatlessness with a story. "We have this friend who is a vegan, and the last time we went out for supper, he kept criticizing what we were eating, telling us what sort of conditions the chickens and cows were living in before they became our supper, how much pollution was caused because of them. I mean, I don't need that shit."

We are hardwired toward the personal. Otherwise there is simply too much information for our bodies and minds to process. Our hearts can go out to, say, the famine-ravaged people of Somalia. Maybe we will even flip out the old credit card and make a donation toward helping them. Alex would do that—she is a good person. But to connect our choice to abstain from eating meat with famine in a country we've never been to filled with people we don't know is a stretch. What is not a stretch is the justifiable annoyance we feel when a friend attacks our choices and uses friendship as a platform for proselytizing, no matter how genuine a place of passionate global engagement they might be coming from.

So what do we do? How do we get individuals, ourselves included, to take seriously the reality that our production of greenhouse gases is strangling our world, and that our simple, everyday choices matter?

The answer might exist in the garden, where a relationship long-severed by the convenience of grocery stores gets reestablished: the relationship between soil and rain and the cycle of life, between manure and death and compost and fertilization, where that fundamental, inarguable relationship between the climate and what we end up eating has a chance of blossoming. The garden is where food becomes personal.

The Garden: Adam and Eve

We began in the Garden. The opening words of the book of Genesis introduce us to God. God is a Creator. Out of chaos and darkness, God shaped order and light. With intentionality, thoughtfulness, and, most importantly, joy and delight, God crafted the complexities of life. *God saw that it was good*—the affirmation runs as God's mantra throughout the whole work of creation. Human beings were formed within the sweeping and expansive web of inspired existence, with one distinction: we are created in the "image and likeness of God." Should we be uncertain of what exactly that means, these verses offer clues. The image of God must have something to do with the ability to create, the capacity for joy, and the purpose of relationship, because what are the days of creation and God's intricate enactment of life but a description of the relationship between the various works God creates, the relationship between Creator and creature?

The verses that subsequently unfold support this assessment of what that divine image means for humankind. Adam was created out of earth. The forming of his body came from the life God had already created. God gave Adam "dominion" over the rest of the created order, trusting him, on behalf of all, with profound responsibility. God asked Adam to participate in the work of creation by naming his fellow creatures. God created Eve out of Adam's own body in order that he might have a partner. *It is not good for man to be alone.* God blessed the man and woman with everything they needed: food, peace, and an intimate relationship with their Maker. They lived in a garden of abundance, flavor, and beauty.

There was something in that garden that was not for them. The Tree of Knowledge of Good and Evil stood in the middle of Eden, and Adam and Eve were forbidden from eating its fruit. It was a reasonable limitation. It was also impossible. They could eat a vast variety of delicious foods, they could have more than enough, *but they could not have everything.* There existed, within the tapestry of life, parts that were not for human consumption, which served another purpose. Adam and Eve claimed it for themselves anyway and ate. God's judgment fit the crime: humankind would work and sweat to produce food. The effortlessness of the Garden that seduced Adam and Eve into thinking that all of God's creation existed merely to provide for human need was now tempered by ongoing physical toil that reminded them not to take for granted that they had life through the gift of other life, that they existed within these patterns of life and had to learn how to honor those relationships, rather than exploit them or attempt to exist outside of them.

The Temptations of Jesus

Jesus began his own ministry by confronting temptations similar to his biblical ancestors. As befits an anointed one of God, Jesus discerned the direction of his public ministry with a time of fasting and purification in the wilderness.

Jesus was tempted toward the same exploitative and forgetful relationship with God's creation that tripped up Adam and Eve. "Turn these rocks into bread," the tempter so reasonably suggested to Jesus. It was not just that eating bread would break Jesus's commitment to fasting. On a more basic level, Jesus would have succumbed to the sin of turning the world around him into nothing more than a resource to be mined for his own satisfaction. Rocks are not bread. Their purpose within God's creation is not to feed us. Jesus passed the test by recognizing that his hunger did not trump God's purpose—not all things existed to serve individual need.[1]

In John's gospel, Jesus's temptation comes full circle in his resurrection. Mary Magdalene, the first witness of the risen Christ, wept in the garden as she came to terms with recent events: Jesus whipped and stripped and hung to die, the last acts of care she and the other women offered to his body before burying him, the inexplicable absence of a body, the empty tomb, strange and holy and disturbing and improbable words. In the midst of her outpouring of sadness and fear, Mary met the gardener. Only when the gardener spoke her name did she recognize him as Jesus.

---

1. Thank you to Dr. Michael Thompson, general secretary of the Anglican Church of Canada, for this insight.

It is not just that she recognizes the gardener as Jesus, however; it is also that she recognized Jesus as the Gardener.

At the outset of this book I talked about how Jesus embodied right relationship with hunger. He identified need and longing at the heart of human life, and, through acts of healing, feeding, redeeming, and forgiving, he pointed the way to a loving relationship with God and a compassionate relationship with one another. The most significant barrier Jesus encountered was the inability of individuals to see their own need, and therefore to see themselves as related to one another. Those who believed their lives were self-made and complete had the hardest time receiving the Good News: "It is easier for a camel to go through the eye of a needle than for someone who is rich to enter the kingdom of God" (Matt. 19:24).

The bigger picture of Jesus's right relationship with hunger was his embodiment of right relationship, period. The garden is where food becomes personal, where we physically encounter the connection between human life and the created order in which we exist with our labor and sweat, where the dirt and the gift of nourishment are respected and understood and cultivated. The biblical witness adds other layers to the gardening image. The Garden is where human beings once found themselves abundantly fed, and where they walked in natural intimacy with their Creator. There is an implicit connection made in the relationship between gardener and land, and gardener and God.

Although John's gospel is the only place in which Jesus is actually described in gardening terms, it sheds light on Jesus's entire ministry. In his disruptive acts of feeding and healing, in his disarming intimacy with Abba God, in his calloused desert-dry hands reaching out to touch lepers and corpses, in his receiving water from a Samaritan woman at a well, in his accepting hospitality from a notorious tax collector, in his anointing by a nameless and extravagant woman just before his death, Jesus revealed himself as one who cultivated, tilled, and nurtured everyone growing in God's garden. Jesus showed us that we meet God in the mud and muck that marks our existence.

Mary was right. Jesus is the Gardener. In the Jewish tradition Jesus followed, and out of the Christian tradition initiated in Jesus's name, we see resonant patterns of living that enable us to claim our right relationship with the land, with God, with one another.

The Living Diet

Reconnecting Body and World

If Alex is emblematic of our lack of care and attention to the environment in the face of catastrophic climate change, then one could argue that our apathy is driven by a perceived lack of personal relationship. We have forgotten how we are personally invested in the world around us. Apathy for our environment also causes problems for us personally, particularly in our disordered relationship with our food and our bodies. We fail to see how our carelessness toward the soil, water, and air makes our bodies unwell. The Living Diet gives us possibilities to reclaim our personal relationship with the world around us. These next practices not only open our hearts to the crucial task of caring for the environment, but also enable the healing of our relationships with our bodies and the food we put into them.

Farmers Market

Everyone in St. Catharines goes to the farmers market. Except me. I've been a couple of times. I love everything about the idea of a farmers market, but my weekend work and family schedule never leave that window of time open long enough for me to get there.

Nonetheless, I get to enjoy the market vicariously through my friends' stories. Local musicians play, many of whom we know through the church. People that I love and care about all run into each other. Delicious homemade local and close-to-local items are bought and sold. A bread-maker responds week by week to customer comments to perfect her recipe for gluten-free bread. For around seven dollars, you can buy three blue-cheese stuffed olives, which I'm told are very good, especially if you like olives. Organic vegetables can be ordered in advance and picked up from one of the vendors. One might criticize this as simply a yuppie, trendy thing for the high-browed foodie culture, but it can't be criticized for much else. Trendy or not, there is something very real, very right about buying food in the context of community, fellowship, entertainment, conversation, and enjoyment. How many people describe going to the grocery store with such glowing accounts?

Community Supported Agriculture Programs (CSA)

I let myself off the hook somewhat for not making it to the market because my family has at times been part of a community supported agriculture program (CSA). Essentially the program allows us to buy a share in a local farm. Each week through the spring and summer, we receive a basket of seasonal produce. Ours included options for egg and meat shares. In Orillia, a few families belonged to the program with us, and we took turns driving out to the farm to pick up our shares. When there, we wandered around to see how things were coming up. We visited with the animals that eventually provided meat for our tables. We saw where the eggs were laid. Our baskets included surprisingly honest cooking notes, like, "Rinse cauliflower in saltwater to get rid of any wormies." It was all organic, and there were some added benefits and challenges that came along with that.

A banner year for Ontario produce was 2013. It was sunny, it was hot, and there were plenty of lush and gentle rains. We had suffered with the farm through a drought the year before, enjoying a significantly reduced harvest in our weekly baskets, the size and shape of the fruits pinched from lack of rain, although the flavor tended to be delightfully rich. Despite the great conditions this next year, we nonetheless found our basket shares meagre. A half of a portion of beans here, a teasing of tomatoes there. At the end of the very puzzling summer, I discovered from our provider what the problem had been. A bug infestation had depleted the farm's produce. "That makes sense," I told her. "In the future, just let us know what's going on. We know it's not a grocery store. We invest in the program because we want to know what's actually happening on a real farm with real food. Just let us know so we understand." I had been agonizing all summer whether to discontinue our participation in the program only to rediscover what I had wanted to learn all along: that there are relationships involved in the food we eat. There is a story behind the bounty we do or don't receive at our tables.

Community Gardens

St. David's began a community garden in the summer of 2011. A small group of parishioners tend the garden through the spring and summer, and midweek summer worship is held in the middle of the cucumbers and tomatoes, followed by a "gardening party" (bring your own spade). Produce is harvested and given to the local food bank, which consistently looks for healthier food options for their clients than canned goods. In 2012, a group from the hospital's mental health program became tenants in the church's garden, using the produce for their own tables and the experience for their own gardening and cooking education. It also had a positive impact on both their mental and physical health. The church gets weekly updates on the number of pounds harvested and donated. And the gardening team keeps looking for ways to extend the work into the hands of more and more people. Regardless of whether you are on the team digging and planting the beds in the spring, or you pick a few weeds as you are walking by, or your kids can't wait to run through after church and pluck some green beans to munch, or if you simply look forward to the updates on how things are growing, the community garden provides an excellent opportunity to forge connection through the blessing of land and the human hands working with that land to produce the miracle of food, connecting shared resources with the shared needs of the community.

Home Gardens

Growing our own food at a community garden or in your own backyard has a ripple effect. We better understand the relationship between soil, sun, water, personal finesse, and downright luck, and the food that is the end result of this peculiar and particular combination of factors. We reclaim choices about what we put into our bodies, independent of the food industry. We invest in creative, organic solutions rather than pesticides, experimenting with the growing factors in our domain of power, and respecting the growing factors outside of our control. We change our attitude toward the food that we continue to buy through the established consumer channels. We make a positive environmental impact by eating as locally as it gets—our own backyard. We create an expanded consciousness around food: the dirt under our fingernails serves as a potent reminder of how clearly the food we eat cannot be reduced to a mere calorie count.

Cooking

> You don't have to worry about the calories or salt if you're prepar-
> ing it yourself. Eighty precent of our salt in the modern diet comes
> from processed food, so if you're making your own, you can be
> very liberal with the salt. You can stop worrying about nutrients if
> you're cooking yourself. Even poor women who cook have health-
> ier diets than rich women who don't cook. It transcends usual
> class bias of the modern diet.
>
> —Michael Pollan[2]

A free pass from worrying about calories and salt? Michael Pollan, in the third installment on his trilogy on eating, writes about the act of home cooking and makes it sound like an awfully good deal for the individual. Although Pollan isn't writing from a religious perspective, it doesn't take him long to address the relational, cultural, and even global implications of preparing our own food. Part of the argument at the heart of *Cooked: A Natural History of Transformation* is that cooking meals from real ingredients is a powerful choice against the food indus-try selling us food that hurts us, made from ingredients that hurt our earth. To give the job of cooking over to the food industry is to change our eating into an antipersonal act; a conglomerate, rather than a per-son, decides what we eat and from where. Cooking, in contrast, is the choice to invest in knowing where our ingredients come from and to stand against an industry standard that layers fat, sugar, and salt onto cheap and overprocessed ingredients that come from far away and were made a long time ago, so that we are fooled into thinking that we are

---

2. Interview with Michael Pollan on CBC Radio Q, June 6, 2013.

eating something delicious. As Pollan states, "Cooking is all about connection, I've learned, between us and other species, other times, other
cultures (human and microbial and both), but, most important, other
people. Cooking is one of the more beautiful forms that human generosity takes. . . . But the very best cooking, I discovered, is also a form
of intimacy."[3]

He gives a good sales pitch, but the question remains: how? The
Living Diet seeks to provide options for people in a variety of circumstances. The reality for many of us is we don't have the time, the skill,
or perhaps the inclination for cooking. I used to love to cook. As I
found myself increasingly worn down by the pickiness of my small
children, my husband's latent cooking skills started to emerge and he
took over primary responsibility in the kitchen. Consider which of the
following categories you might fall into, and what type of solution you
might be seeking:

1. **You love to cook,** but you have limited time or picky children.
   You can easily slip into too many dinners out, or be too read-
   ily tempted by tater tots and frozen pizzas. Make an effort to
   surround yourself with people who enjoy cooking, who will
   exchange recipes and enthusiasm. Spend Saturday mornings gab-
   bing while you make casseroles for the week and laugh (rather
   than cry) about what pantry staple your children have decided
   they won't eat any more. Plan social cooking time with your kids
   to teach them the same sorts of kitchen skills taught to you. I
   am part of a monthly Gourmet Group with a group of friends.
   My daughter's curiosity is piqued by the recipes I prepare to take
   out with me, which then translates into her willingness to try
   making one of the new dishes with me at another time for our
   family. In other words, if you love to cook and don't have time,
   combine cooking with socializing downtime that will nourish
   not only your family's stomachs, but also your mind and emotions and soul.

---

3. Pollan, *Cooked*, 415.

2. **You would *like* to love to cook.** Despite the plethora of gourmet cooking shows, not to mention the exotic ingredients that have suddenly become available at most local supermarkets for only modestly astronomical prices, basic cooking skills are a lost art. I would recommend the aforementioned *Cooked* as well as *The Supper of the Lamb* by Robert Farrar Capon to both inspire and teach some basic knowledge in the whys and wherefores of kitchen chemistry. Of course, you can sign up for a cooking class. Many local grocery stores offer them in their community kitchen facilities. But given the relational argument at the heart of *The Living Diet*, you can go one better than cooking class and seek out an acquaintance with some time and skill. Faith communities are a great place to identify someone who fits this bill and ask them to mentor you in the kitchen. What are some of their time-tested recipes? What are the basic ratios and ingredients for salad dressings and roux? What are pantry staples? And what do they recommend for picky eaters? There is no better way to learn the love of cooking than through the sharing of stories and experiences and the testing, tasting, tweaking, and teaching of recipes.

3. **You don't want to cook.** You have as much interest in cooking as I have in learning to wax floors. It's okay. You can still change your relationship with food and participate in this most important part of the Living Diet. You just need to choose a thoughtful approach to convenience food.

   a) *Use summer as a free pass.* Ontario has a four to five month growing season. If you live somewhere with a longer one, consider yourself lucky. But even here, up to 40 percent of the year can be a free pass on cooking. Just let the fresh tastes of summer do all of the work. Eat asparagus through June, green beans and sweet peas in July, corn and peaches in August and into September, slice up tomatoes and throw some fresh basil and salt and pepper on them, and once you scare up a protein and throw a potato or two in the microwave, you've got fresh, local, great-tasting food without ever having to do more than boil some water and locate the salt, pepper, and butter.

b) *Choose convenience food wisely.* For the rest of the year, or where fresh and local may be harder to come by, depending on your geography, spend some time getting acquainted with your grocery store conveniences. Canned and frozen foods might not be hugely flavorful, but sometimes it is easier to find items in these areas of the store that at least are not imported. With some care, you can honor the relationship with the world around you through the convenience foods you buy. Likewise, things like prepackaged lettuce, canned tomatoes, and frozen veggies can save you time and hassle, while also caring for the relationship you have with your body by choosing conveniences which skip the salt-sugar-fat smorgasbord.

c) *Make friends.* The best choice for the Living Diet, even if you hate cooking, is to develop a relationship with someone who cooks. Don't worry, I'm not suggesting you should marry someone for their culinary skills, although, as far as arranged marriages go, it's not a bad consideration. Scout out someone in your faith community or neighborhood who knows how to cook and has time. Perhaps it is even someone on a fixed income or pension who would be pleased to make a few extra dollars. Use the bonds of friendship and community to arrange for convenience food outside of the reach of the food industry. You can funnel your "eating out" money to your newfound friendship. They, in turn, can prepare a weekly assortment of casseroles, soups, or stews. You get all of the benefits of homemade, and you can remain that person who hates cooking.

Ethical Meat

In the Hindu tradition, followers are encouraged to refrain from meat, alcohol, garlic, radishes, and onions—all of which are seen as intrinsically harmful to the interior life. (A life without garlic?) It assumes a spiritual understanding of the food we eat. For example, if an animal is killed violently or the attitude of the person cooking is negative, it creates particular vibrations within the food and those vibrations have a spiritual and emotional impact on those consuming it.[4]

Maybe you are not vegan or vegetarian. I admire and respect those who are, but I am not there. Or I'm not there right now. Even within the domain of meat-eating though, we can make substantially different choices.

I give thanks for CSA program meat and egg shares. I give thanks for those farmers I have met through the church or through my kids' piano lesson group who give me the opportunity to stock my freezer with local beef and chicken. I give thanks because I see and hear the respect and care with which they both raise and slaughter their animals. It is my responsibility to use the parts of the animal to the fullest extent possible, and to do so with gratitude.

Veganism and Vegetarianism

Many of those who are most connected to the world around them, who feel most strongly the responsibility we bear for our environment and our fellow creatures, make the choice to abstain from eating meat. It is a generous and thoughtful choice. Whereas it might be the case that all human beings could exist in a balanced relationship of careful and modest consumption of other animals, the fact is that industries that promote meat-eating are choking the planet, not to mention causing large numbers of animals to live in the most deplorable of circumstances throughout their short and abused lives. At the very least, practitioners of the Living Diet should consider looking for opportunities to eat less meat. Consider a few possibilities:

- Commit to eating meatless meals when in restaurants. Since everyone is ordering their own food anyway, your vegetarian choice does not further complicate the choices available at the shared supper table.
- Go meatless one day a week. Devout Catholics, for example, refrain from eating meat on Fridays. And there is a bonus: even occasional vegetarianism has an impact on reducing your grocery bill.

---

4. Funk, *Thoughts Matter*, 29.

- The forty-day season of Lent is a great time to abstain from meat-eating. It is challenging and meaningful, without being a daunting lifelong commitment.

If I cannot currently abstain from eating meat completely, I can maintain the utmost respect for those who choose vegetarianism or veganism. That might mean having to deal with some guilt. My friend Alex was understandably annoyed by her vegan friend who nattered at her about the conditions in which the chicken on her plate was bred and slaughtered. Nobody likes to feel bad about their food choices midconsumption. Alex's experience isn't uncommon. There is a stereotype associated with non-meat-eaters which suggests that they are irritatingly preachy. They look down their nose at those of us who haven't got the fortitude to make similarly generous choices for the life of our fellow creatures and the life of the planet. The truth of the matter, however, is that our veggie friends might not be preachy at all. We might just feel guilty because deep down, we know they are right.

The Living Diet invites us to react to another's thoughtful and conscientious food choices, not with irritation, but with gratitude for the challenge and conversation that come with being asked to consider our choices more deeply.

Lord of the Feast

Consider this: Soylent is a food substitute, available since 2014, that is designed to fully nourish an individual without having to actually eat real food. Although it sounds like science-fiction—and in fact, it cheekily takes its name from a fictional invention[1]—the appeal of what it promises is undeniable:

Soylent—Free Your Body
What if you never had to worry about food again?

For anyone who struggles with allergies, heartburn, acid reflux or digestion, has trouble controlling weight or cholesterol, or simply doesn't have the means to eat, well, Soylent is for you.

Soylent frees you from the time and money spent shopping, cooking and cleaning, puts you in excellent health, and vastly reduces your environmental impact by eliminating much of the waste and harm coming from agriculture, livestock, and food-related trash.[2]

Food without the fuss. Eating without cooking. A meal on the run freed not only from all of the typical fast-food drawbacks, but from all of the other food problems as well (hormones, allergens, unethical proteins, lack of time, lack of money, waste). Those who consume

---

1. The inventor named it after a fictional food from the novel *Make Room! Make Room!* on which the 1973 film *Soylent Green* was loosely based.

2. *https://www.bluegartr.com/threads/119664-Soylent-What-if-You-Never-Had-to-Worry-About-Food-Again-(People-Not-Included)*.

it instead of food report clearer thinking, better skin, more energy, and . . . wait for it . . . weight loss.

The appeal of Soylent is undeniable. It promises everything that we believe we so desperately crave: more time, better skin, thinner body. It eliminates the stress of not only having to prepare and eat food but also removes the difficult work of deciding what we will put into our bodies. The mere invention of Soylent is indicative of just how much cultural dis-ease there is around eating.

When my now-husband popped the question, I told him I was marrying him for his money. Dan knew I was kidding—he was a broke student at the time. In fact, the joke was a cover-up for the real reason I fell for him: he was not afraid of food.

Okay, so maybe I'm still partly joking. But only partly. When we met, I was still a prisoner of my own particular set of food anxieties. Thankfully, I could nonetheless identify, be attracted to, and reach out toward another possibility. I knew I wanted to create a home, start a family, and raise children with a partner who enjoyed eating. As we began to plan our future together, it was the warm and bustling kitchen and a large and merry dining room table that settled into my imagination as the key pieces of what would be our new life together.

Although the millions to whom Soylent is being marketed might claim to love food and judge a modern-day "dream home" by the lavishness of its kitchen, the regular event of eating remains shrouded in fear.

Fear of *Real* Food

From Soylent to TV dinners to packaged cookie dough and minute rice dishes, the modern food industry provides all kinds of ways to cut corners and opt for something food-like rather than the real thing. Although we have become almost entirely sold on the notion that we do not have the time or skill to invest in food preparation, these seemingly amazing culinary inventions fail to actually give people extra time. We opt for more and more convenience, yet we become further stretched. We treat meals as an inconvenience to be effectively managed, rather than an opportunity for refreshing, gathering, delighting, and giving thanks.

Fear of Calories

My stomach is not as limber as it once was. I do have to make choices about what I will refrain from eating so that I can enjoy an extra course, a bigger meal, or a special dessert. But it saddens me that "indulging" has become a dirty word. The meal as a celebration of taste, texture, color, ritual, and tradition—the menu chosen because of how flavors pair with one another, the memories evoked by particular foods, the delight and challenge of creating and serving dishes that have been carefully prepared and brought together to form an overall experience—is relegated almost entirely to reality TV cooking shows and expensive Michelin-star restaurants. Cooking has become a spectator sport. Gourmet cooking, in that rarefied circle of celebrity chefs, elicits minute praise for and critique of every detail of the food's composition. As much as I love cooking shows, they have evolved into a bizarre combination of celebrating the details of food creation, while also sidelining the audience from being able to participate in the most important part of the meal: eating. It troubles me to see the judges walk away from each beautifully prepared plate, leaving it sampled yet mostly uneaten, reinforcing wastefulness, even as they elevate and admire culinary prowess.

Yet, for all of the growing "foodie culture" seen on television and in our ever-expanding grocery stores, an awkwardness to our actual consumption remains. It would be considered poor form to attend a concert and then comment throughout the performance that you should really be home doing housework, that the evening of fun was keeping you from vacuuming and is therefore responsible for ruining your carpets. It is somehow acceptable, however, to sit at a meal that has taken the host an entire day to prepare and discuss whose diet has been broken by the meal, what sort of punishing adjustments will have to be made over the coming days in order to make up for the indulgence, or to apologetically insist, "Oh, just a small amount for me." Meanwhile, the delights at hand become invisible: for example, homemade bread fresh out of the oven, real aged parmesan cheese liberally sprinkled on the salad, a dessert made from scratch and full of things like eggs and butter and vanilla. The offering of the meal is rejected by the worry we have learned to bring with us to every plate.

Fear of Thinking

When my eating was at its most obsessive, I hid in my room studying with my hand in a comforting bag of Doritos. "I just love food too much," I would say out loud when skirting around the edges of my problem. Eating a whole bag of salty fried food alone while doing philosophy homework is not a portrait of someone who loves food, but of one choosing to eat rather than think.

Although it is rare to host a dinner party where the guests allow themselves guilt-free enjoyment, it is common practice to scarf take-out on the run, to stuff packaged cookies into our mouths because they happen to be available, and to treat eating as a thoughtless, or worse, covert activity—an indulgence to be denied or hidden and to be engaged in alone.

❉ ❉ ❉

I married Dan for his stomach, and I have often been disappointed by the lack of eating enthusiasm from our invited dinner guests. My observations may sound like they boil down to problems of a merely personal nature: ego (my culinary skills not adequately affirmed), preference (my choosing a mate who can join me in enjoying the kitchen and the table), or maybe loneliness (finding far too few kindred "stomachs" in my circle of friends). However, I understand these fears intimately. I have fallen prey to each of them. I know what it is to be afraid of food. Being scared of eating is not just a personal problem, it is a collective one. And the consequences of our collective fear are not just physical, but also, and primarily, spiritual.

A Feast

Dan and I have a favorite way of ringing in a new year. Charles Inn in Niagara-on-the-Lake offers a December 31st extravaganza: a seven-course, three-and-a-half-hour meal. We invite friends who we know will enjoy the evening. We dress up. We strategize. After all, this behemoth of a supper follows on the heels of at least three weeks of nonstop Christmas baking, special family dinners, evenings out, and a fridge all-too-temptingly full of wonderful things to eat.

I pride myself in having a large appetite, and given that the meal doesn't begin until after 9 p.m. (perfectly timed so that dessert is just beginning when the ball drops), and although I should know better, I usually stampede into the first course with far too much bravado. Seven courses seem like nothing when your stomach has been holiday stretched and you are so hungry that becoming full doesn't feel like any sort of realistic possibility. About three courses in, I am humbled. Making it through all of the meal with appreciation for the detail of each carefully prepared course, without wasting any of the beautifully prepared dishes or missing out on the intricacy of the relationship of color, texture, and flavor built into each food and wine pairing is no easy feat.

Salad progresses to soup, which unfolds into a fish ragout, then a lobster tail and tenderloin, rounded out with cheese and chocolate. It is a stunning culinary journey. Each person in our dinner party invariably struggles to find new corners in their stomachs where the next bite might fit. All of us eat too much. And not one of us would suggest that it is the kind of eating in which we should regularly indulge; once a year is about right for both stomach and budget. Yet this offers the perfect way of ending one year and beginning a new one, and this extraordinary meal has a lesson to teach, entirely transferrable to our regular, everyday eating.

Counter to our world of fearful eating stands the witness of *The Feast*. God has created a world of taste and texture, of extraordinary flavor and unending diversity. Built into the fabric of our survival is the capacity for joy and love. Eating, whether the most elaborate or the simplest of dishes, is inherently enjoyable and social—a gift that draws people together and makes our hearts glad.

Yet we deny our very nature and turn away from the gift of offering and receiving hospitality. We isolate ourselves from one another and turn our bodies and spirits into warring entities pitted against one another in a battle of competing desires. Too often we opt either for some culturally validated story of restraint or for stuffing our faces, when both extremes mask the ways in which life feels out of our control. We choose neither restraint nor indulgence, but alienation.

My New Year's Eve experience wasn't about overeating. It was about reclaiming something that is as important to remember when eating noodles and salad at home with my family as it is when I'm decked out in our formal wear, eating the creations of a top chef. Feasting is about slowing down the pace of life and paying attention to the details. It is about indulging in beauty and receiving the gift of food and all that goes with it: laughter, conversation, renewed relationships and spirits.

Lord of the Feast

> On this mountain the LORD of hosts will make for all peoples
>> a feast of rich food, a feast of well-matured wines,
>> of rich food filled with marrow, of well-matured wines
>>> strained clear.
> And he will destroy on this mountain
>> the shroud that is cast over all peoples,
>> the sheet that is spread over all nations;
> he will swallow up death for ever.
> Then the Lord GOD will wipe away the tears from all faces,
>> and the disgrace of his people he will take away
>>> from all the earth,
>> for the LORD has spoken.
>
> (Isa. 25:6–8)

When Jesus began his public ministry, he wasn't as much of an ascetic as people expected. He noted, in the face of his critics, that when John the Baptist refrained from food and drink, they criticized him. Yet, when Jesus came, eating and drinking, he was criticized as well (Matt. 11:18–19). He should have been more holy, more reserved, if he wanted to be taken seriously as a teacher and prophet of God.

The complaint against Jesus, however, was a thinly veiled concern, not about the fact that he enjoyed eating and drinking, but *who he was with*. Priest and theologian Donald Schell notes that Jesus feasted intentionally, in a way that specifically picked up the eschatological imagery of the prophet Isaiah: the meal was a way of drawing together people of all races and backgrounds, of revealing the fulfillment of people who were called to share together in God's good gifts, and discover that the power of death and sorrow had been eliminated. Jesus's prophetic sign of "enacting God's feast and welcoming all—especially unprepared sinners"—was the "scandal and offense," in fact, that results in Jesus's death.[3]

I have discussed Jesus's use of food as a way of inviting people into relationship with God, noting that he didn't come up with this imagery himself, but learned it from his people. The Jewish faith is laden with instances where God reaches out to the people through manna, fresh springs of water, a land flowing with milk and honey, and through a call to remember and celebrate God's blessings by participating in a regular pattern of seasonal feasts.

Nonetheless, the centrality of the feast in Jesus's teaching led to surprise and alarm. In John's gospel, Jesus's first miracle was the changing of water into wine. *On the third day* . . . the account begins. We know from the introduction that what is being described has not only a temporal dimension, but also an eternal one. *On the third day* there was a wedding feast, and when the wine ran out Jesus provided for the continuation of the party. This is wine that is of such quality that the already well-lubricated guests take note. They praised their host for saving the best for last.

The miracle is scandalous in its frivolity for some, yet, as Jesus's life unfolded, we can see it was consistent with Jesus's emphasis on the feast: in meals with sinners and outcasts, his feeding of the thousands with fish and bread, his breaking bread in the upper room on his last night, his resurrection appearances, and the banquet imagery that he chose time and again in his teaching. He invited his followers to imagine the offering of God as one that brought joy to bellies and hearts and disrupted "business as usual."

Food is a sign of God's loving care for us. It is also a sign that the track we are on is a significant distance away from God's. The prophetic sign of the feast issues an invitation both to repent and to rejoice. The lost art of feasting in our world today is a sign of an intense spiritual dislocation, not just from the possibility of who God invites us to be, but from the basic nature of what it is to be human. When we do not know how to feast, how to step outside of the ordinary and be extraordinary with one another, we risk closing ourselves off from the variety

---

3. Donald Schell, "Discerning Open Table in Community and Mission," *ATR* 94, no. 2, (2012): 251.

of flavors and blessings God has woven into the world. In contrast, when we rediscover how to share those gifts with thought, care, attentiveness, story, and thanksgiving, we taste something of our capacity to live with one another in peace and for "the shroud that is cast over all peoples" (Isa. 25:7) to be lifted. We also change our relationship with food, erasing the lines so strongly etched against our bodies and ourselves by the deep-seated fear we have learned. We can abide in the joy and gratitude central in the feast.

The Living Diet

Feasting

The Living Diet embraces and reclaims the lost art of the feast. We set aside regular time for sharing in a meal where we drop our defenses with our relationship with food. When we find the courage to declare a truce in our war on food, food responds with a gracious yielding of riches. But what makes a feast? And how can even those who are too busy, too strapped for cash, or too lost in the kitchen participate?

No Calorie Counting

I wonder about the damage done when we translate our relationship with food into numbers. I admit that calorie counting has only ever backfired on me, and anecdotally I would report that I have seen very few weight loss strategies that are based on a mathematical formula of restraint and denial work in the long-term. Although I notice an unhelpful reductionism in how we view food when we label everything with a calorie count, I also understand that keeping track of how much we put into our bodies is a cornerstone of dietary advice. I am not a fan of counting calories. I am also not a dietician.

In feasting, however, there is no room for counting calories. We need to train our collective consciousness away from phrases like "this will go right to my hips," or "I'll have to starve myself for the next three days to make up for this" when we share a meal. This recalibration of language takes time, however. Those who are serious about reimagining how they think and talk about food might consider getting silly. A lighthearted game around the supper table is a way of beginning to be aware of the language we use. Give everyone a pin or a coin. Make a list of taboo words: calorie, diet, weight, waistline, gluten, etc. If someone at the table catches another using one of the outlawed words, they get to take that individual's pin or coin. The laughter generated by a little friendly competition creates space for talking differently about the food we put into our bodies.

Pig Out?

Feasting doesn't mean eating to the point of sickness or discomfort. All-you-can-eat buffets, for example, need to be approached with care. Individually loading up my plate with what I individually want for a no-holds-barred take-down to "get my money's worth" without heeding any signal of fullness that my body will inevitably send out usually ends up looking far more like mindless eating than embracing the beautiful gift of food. That being said, we have a favorite buffet place we go to with a favorite friend, where our endless conversation and great joy in seeing one another stretches out the meal into a leisurely, laughter-filled time. Feasting need not lead to sickness. Food should be enjoyed with ample time for digestion, all the while attentive to our body's responses to the good food that has been prepared.

Guests

My friend Cheryl told me about being invited with her two girls to a BBQ at her friend Kitty's house. Kitty is known for being a generous host, and Cheryl's daughters enjoyed the evening. Several weeks later, Cheryl was driving one of her daughters to an after-school activity when she called out from the back seat, "Hey, that guy was at Kitty's barbeque!" "That guy" was walking in downtown St. Catharines with all of his worldly goods piled in a shopping cart. He was a homeless man whom Kitty had met through our church's breakfast program. She invited him to her party.

Whether you sit down with family, friends, or those you would like to know better, whether a small number or a great number, or even if it is just you and your significant other, the most important part of the feast is the people with whom you share it. The Meal is one of God's great instruments for forging, strengthening, and rebuilding relationships, as well as breaking down barriers between us that often seem insurmountable.

Allergies

The list of allergies, intolerances, and special dietary needs that so many live with is staggering. A few of my friends are made so ill by common foods—dairy, eggs, corn, wheat, peanuts, or almonds—that they feel forced into antisocial postures. Their food has to be prepared with such militant care that there are few places they can go to enjoy a meal. In the world in which we now live, a critical part of hosting a feast is inquiring about dietary needs or allergies *ahead* of time as we figure out what to serve. When we embrace feasting, figuring out how to include those who otherwise find it hard to eat with others becomes an opportunity for an extra level of generosity and thoughtfulness in our meal planning and preparation.

Ambience

I like to create a special playlist and set the table with a brightly colored tablecloth. If I can talk Dan into washing it later, the china and silverware we received as wedding presents come out as well. Beyond that, ambience is not my forte. Dan is the one who lights the candles, decorates the house for the seasons, and often suggests getting a bouquet of flowers to distribute into small arrangements around the house. No matter your skill level in this department, the idea is to recognize that what you eat is only one part of extending hospitality.

Limited Technology

Oftentimes the playlist I create for an occasion never ends up getting turned on, or it is playing at such a low level that it is barely heard. I like putting special care into the music shared, but in doing so, I am reminded that the conversation at the feast is most important. Put your own phone on silent while sharing a meal with others. Invite guests to turn off their devices. If you are a household that regularly has the television on, turn it off for a few hours. Limit the use of technology and wade into the life-giving waters of person-to-person interaction. Then, try to carry these same boundaries into your regular mealtimes as well.

Connection

The feast is meant to connect us to a larger story. Throughout history, feasting has been part of religious practice. The annual and weekly religious feasts of Jesus's people were the glue that bound them together and kept them close to the story of God's faithful presence in their lives. They followed specific instructions for what was to take place when they gathered for special meals.

In our predominantly secular world, where the company around our North American tables is quite likely to be religiously mixed, there are other simple ways of connecting the food we eat to a story that is bigger than filling our stomachs. Although your guests might have a variety of feelings about religion, most grown-ups have been trained to be respectful of the traditions of others. A quick explanation that in your faith tradition you give thanks before a meal, followed by a simple prayer of gratitude before people dig in, is minimally awkward, and potentially profound in the effect it creates. À la secular North American Thanksgiving feast, you might also take a moment to invite your guests to name aloud something for which they are grateful, even if your particular meal falls outside the bounds of the holiday. Gratitude connects our food to a bigger picture than just scarfing down our "just desserts."

For Noncooks

I said that there would be flexibility built into the Living Diet. So what about noncooks? What about those who are too busy to host a feast? There are many for whom the intricacies of cookbook reading, menu planning, grocery shopping, and top-chefing fall far outside the realm of feasibility. I make no pretensions about my prowess, but I have been known to love puttering in the kitchen. Nonetheless, there are many weeks when the thought of having to scrape together enough hours to prepare a meal for anyone other than our immediate family is utterly exhausting. Beyond the crunch of schedules, there are many who have only the faintest idea of how to go about cooking from scratch, and some have little to no desire to learn. I can relate. I feel the same way about dusting.

If you fall into this category, don't worry. You can still initiate a feast. One of our family friends always says that her favorite thing to make for supper is reservations. If you have the means, consider hosting a feast by inviting friends to join you at a carefully selected local restaurant. Give consideration to picking a place where the music won't overpower your ability to talk and where waiters won't be shooting you dirty looks if you linger over dessert. (Rome is a good place . . .) I know very few people who have the financial means to pick up the tab on a regular or even one-off basis. Among our friends, however, is a tacit understanding that we will go "dutch." Perhaps the act of generosity that comes from hosting is missing, but the other elements of connection, gratitude, of entering into a different sort of frame of mind, of enjoying food that has been prepared with a level of thoughtfulness and care are all still possible.

If hosting in your home is an important element for you—and there is something particularly meaningful about doing so—there are still options. We have invited a group of people over on a Sunday afternoon for a directed pot-luck event, asking each household to bring something specific. We were able to enjoy one another's company in a way that would have been next to impossible if we had to prepare the entire meal ourselves. Buying food or drink from a local artisan or farmers market can make the food special and personal, even if you didn't make it. There is something lovely about serving food that has a story attached to it. Dan and I like to tell people which local Ontario winery we picked the wine from, perhaps with a note about the conversations we had with the owner or the wine steward, or how we were able to slip away for a few hours, leaving our kids with their grandmother, so we could get the wine.

If an entire meal is just too much of an undertaking, invite people over for dessert, or wine and cheese. A small and intentional event can be just as powerful in forging new relationships between people.

chapter

14

Fasting—Food as Compassion

Those who observe the day, observe it in honor of the Lord. Also
those who eat, eat in honor of the Lord, since they give thanks to
God; while those who abstain, abstain in honor of the Lord and
give thanks to God. We do not live to ourselves, and we do not die
to ourselves. If we live, we live to the Lord, and if we die, we die to
the Lord; so then, whether we live or whether we die, we are the
Lord's. (Rom. 14:6–8)

This chapter might feel like an about-face from the last one, the
art of the feast, where we discussed our need to push back against
a culture that treats food as an enemy rather than a gift. Fasting
appears to be a denial of this gift. Not eating is the opposite of eating,
right? And yet, fasting is one of the traditional ways in which people
of faith draw closer to God. In fact, fasting is a spiritual practice of all
major world religions; it is both ancient and cross-cultural. And across
all of those traditions, fasting can be seen, not as denying food as a gift,
but as an important means by which that gift is embraced.

Christian monastics observe a regular fast, which is to say they follow a sensible and gentle pattern of consumption: eat only at meals,
eat slowly, eat what is provided, stop when you are full. The average
Christian, on the other hand, is more typically going to encounter the
practice of fasting during the season of Lent.

The forty days of Lent are modeled after Jesus's time of fasting
in the wilderness, following his baptism and prior to beginning his
public ministry. Other religious traditions also uphold great spiritual

129

masters who went through long periods without food. Lenten fasting takes many forms: giving up chocolate or alcohol, limiting meat, cutting back on junk, spending less on treats, and even non-food-related actions like refraining from television or videogames, or deciding to buy only fair-traded or local-sourced items. When people of faith take on these disciplines, we are encouraged to notice how it feels, what it means, how we are freed, and how we are limited. How does being hungry expand my compassion for those who are hungry through no choice of their own? When I spend less on take-out coffee and fast-food lunches, how is that money freed up for other things? On what other things might I, out of compassion, spend that money? Does my body feel different when I notice more carefully what I put into it?

Our family has often given up buying meat and drinking alcohol during Lent. Vegetarianism is a traditional way of observing Lent because the season usually coincides with nature's season for procreation. We give up eating meat as a response to the needs of God's created order, in order to let the natural world regenerate. I enjoy a glass of wine with dinner a few times a week. Going without wine is a discipline that feels consequential. I miss the ease with which I can unwind at the end of the day because of that glass of wine. I miss the heightened enjoyment of food without a rich red to complement the flavors. These small limitations have provided fruitful reflection:

- It is difficult, and somewhat embarrassing to explain to people outside of my immediate family why I am not indulging. It feels inhospitable and antisocial to not share with friends and guests in a glass of wine, to not offer a prime cut of meat at our dinner table.

- I am accustomed to having what I want, when I want it.

- We live in a culture that is accepting of restraint for the sake of self—cutting back in order to lose weight or to be more healthy—but that is puzzled by restraint for the sake of the other—the environment, the animals, the poor.

- Choosing not to have something that I *can* have is an act of freedom. It is difficult. It cuts against the grain of two of the messages I hear most often: *you deserve it, you earned it.* And there is something deeply liberating about restraint that helps me realize that mindless consumption is so naturally and frequently my modus operandi.

The Christian faith upholds feasting and fasting, not as opposites, but as a necessary pair in the joyful, grateful, generous rhythm of the life to which God invites us. It joins other faith traditions in noticing that living a pattern of celebration and indulgence, in combination with thoughtful and intentional restraint, creates an essential balance against all of the ways in which we can become accustomed to consuming that which does not nourish, alienating ourselves from the needs of the world around us, and letting the flavors of life pass us by. Both practices teach us once again that food matters; that food is a gift that deserves to be treated with respect, care, and gratitude; that what we eat and how we eat directly affects our physical, spiritual, and emotional selves; that what we eat and how we eat are acts of relationship and have the power to either strengthen or deny our connection with the rest of creation.

Addiction/Allergy/Intolerance

I kick myself when I host a dinner party and have forgotten to check with my guests about food allergies ahead of time. Although I am annoyed by diet talk at my dinner table, I do want to be understanding of the real struggles that people encounter while seeking joy in eating. Am I conscious of the celiac? Am I aware of the alcoholic? Both examples are not about individual preference but are the difference between health and illness. A person in recovery may find it difficult to even be in a home where wine is present, let alone in a social situation where wine is being consumed. Those who have been diagnosed celiac generally describe a major life revelation, even resurrection, when finally given the reason for feeling sick and crazy all the time. As their damaged gut begins the long and slow process of healing, even a trace amount of gluten can set them off course.

It isn't just when having guests that I have to adjust my thinking around what I serve at the table. I do try to be firm about a "take it or leave it" policy when my cooking is met by the pickiness of my children (although sometimes in the face of yet another meal left untouched by either child, my resolve wears down). That being said, each of us in our family has various reactions to off-kilter eating, particularly when too much sugar creeps into our meals: headaches, back problems, fatigue, irritability, and digestive issues, to name a few. When we better pay attention to the signals our bodies send, we generally feel more energized and clear-minded. When birthday season or Christmas, for example, find us indulging more than usual, we can all easily fall into a sort of addictive spiral—the sugars or refined starches trick our bodies into craving more, even as we feel worse.

Addiction

A glass of wine with supper, a cold beer on a summer's evening, a few drinks with friends on a night off—these are true pleasures of life and a seamless part of the socializing many of us are able to enjoy. However, this simple joy for many of us can turn to inner warfare for others:

- Floodgate Syndrome—one drink leads to an uncontrollable flow of many drinks.
- Isolation—the substance which begins as a lubricant for socializing eventually comes to draw the individual out and cut them off from relationships around them.
- Justification/rationalization—the disease works very effectively in smart people, people who can find numerous and highly creative ways of explaining and encouraging their own destructive behavior.

Alcohol, in any quantity, simply cannot be part of the life of an alcoholic who wishes to no longer destroy her own life. And although there are many other substances to which human beings can get addicted, alcohol is one of the most nuanced and challenging because it is such an acceptable and prevalent part of our collective life.

When my own relationship with food was at its most desperate, I felt like an addict. The idea of food addiction is controversial, although gaining ground in some circles. The thing that seemed most unmanageable to me at the time was the fact that I had to eat. Unlike booze or cocaine, I literally need food to live. But my eating controlled me. Bulimia became my justification, my coping mechanism and my excuse for using food to try and fill (always unsuccessfully) that feeling of emptiness.

A Story of Holy Sacrifice

In the dark, in-between hours of the dead of night, a man prayed in a cold and lonely garden, his prayer acting like an assault on his body, cutting into him like a knife until his tears are blood. His friends succumbed to the fear of the night and chose the forgetfulness of sleep.

"Take this cup of suffering from my lips," he pleaded. He had recently passed a cup of wine among these fair-weather friends, speaking words of covenant: "This is my blood, shed for you. When you drink it, remember me." His words rang with the familiar Jewish temple imagery of sacrifice. Jesus shifted the focus of the sacrifice, however, from the lamb they would have eaten at a Passover supper, to himself. How natural, how human, that he would have second thoughts. There was still time for escape into the quiet countryside, time to abandon the claims he had made of God's new possibility.

"And yet, not my will, but yours be done" was his final surrendering prayer, as his betrayal was at hand. The cup of suffering would not pass from his lips. Jesus's death was revealed, not as murder, not as execution, but as sacrifice because of the Passover meal that preceded it, because of the words of covenant Jesus spoke over the meal.[1] Christians continue to speak of Jesus's death as an offering that gathers all human sin into God's forgiveness, all suffering into God's healing presence.

The Cross

The Cross leads somewhere. The story doesn't end with death, but continues into the surprising Sunday words, "He is risen!" That pattern of death and new life are foundational to describing and shaping the Christian journey. Jesus's call to take up our cross and follow resonated with his earliest followers. The road to new life followed the path of suffering. We will be imprisoned in lies and fear if our lives are simply about avoiding suffering. On the other hand, the suffering we encounter because we have chosen to embrace compassionate love, because we have refused to hide the truth, because we have opened ourselves to the

---

1. Brant Pitre, *The Jewish Roots of the Eucharist* (New York: Random House, 2011), 45.

transformative union with God to which Jesus bears witness, will liberate us for resurrection life.

Eucharist

In the Jewish spirituality of Jesus's day, the sacrifices of the temple did not end with killing an animal, but in eating it. Jewish families made a pilgrimage to the temple in Jerusalem for Passover so that their family's lamb could be slaughtered by the priests, and then the family would gather together at Friday sundown to eat that lamb. Sacrifice included meal.

The Passover Jesus celebrated with his disciples was not simply about remembering Israel's journey from slavery into freedom; it was about *participating* in that journey. As Jesus instituted a new Passover, identifying himself with the Passover lamb, he invited his followers not just to remember him, but to share *in* him. We are not just to think well of Jesus and tell his story, we are to take his life into our own.

As a priest, there are occasional worship opportunities when I am not the one giving out the bread and wine at communion. I love to sit in the chancel of the church, sing the hymns, and open my eyes to what is taking place. I see my beloved church family coming forward with hands open. I know something of their stories: what they hope and pray for, who they have lost, what scars they bear, the worries and sicknesses that weigh them down, the courage and faithfulness that lift them up. They have shared with me moments of suffering and encounters with joy; I have buried their partners and baptized their babies; I have prayed with them in hospital; I have heard their descriptions of why they pray, and how that has transformed their lives. I have encountered their stubbornness and their kindness, their limitedness and their wisdom, their abundant and occasionally hurtful flaws and their deep beauty.

In those quiet moments, I am moved to tears. Whether or not they would use these words to describe their experience, these people know what it is to participate in the dying and rising of Christ. They have drunk from the cup of suffering and they have experienced resurrection. They have somehow taken on the habit of bringing their whole selves to this meal, this sacrifice, and allowed themselves to be shaped and formed by the pattern of Christ.

Back to Food

What does this have to do with food? Allergies, addictions? The wide
variety of acquiescence we have to make in our relationship with food
and our hospitality to one another?

The Book of Common Prayer states the Confession of Sin in these
words: "We have done those things which we ought not to have done.
We have not done those things which we ought to have done. And
there is no health in us."[2]

Mostly these words ring as discordant with today's churchgoer
who rejects such a depraved view of humanity. Sin needs to be balanced with an understanding of human goodness, blessing, and
potential, one might protest. However, if we are attentive, perhaps
we can hear the words resonating with experience. We *do* know what
it is to have our mistakes and our limited human perspective, as well
as our susceptibility to disease and harm, create repercussions for
our own health and well-being, not to mention for the health and
well-being of others around us, or the generations to come. Addiction is a disease that works through basic human pleasure in order
to break down, isolate, and destroy; it takes the things in which we
are meant to delight and turns them into poison. We know that our
misuse of God's creation—our literal "man-handling" of systems of
life that exist in delicate and wondrous balance, the dark blinders we
wear in adjusting or tinkering with the web of life purely based on
our own short-term ability to gain from doing so—has serious and
lasting repercussions. It is theorized that food allergies are symptoms
of all that we have done to upset that balance. Greenhouse gases, polluted waterways, oil spills, plastics, and mercury making their way
into animal and plant life, the proliferation of both antibiotics and
super bugs, overflowing landfills—ever since we tasted the forbidden
fruit and were kicked out of the Garden, we have had trouble keeping
our hands off of what is not ours.

Whether I am an alcoholic, a celiac, or a citizen wondering
where these alarming environmental realities are taking us, I bear that

2. "Morning Prayer," *The Book of Common Prayer 1962 Canada* (Toronto: Anglican Book
Centre, 1962), 4–5.

brokenness in the body that comes forward with hands outstretched to participate in Christ's life and death through communion.

I was wondering out loud to my husband a few years ago about providing an alcohol-free wine at our church's eucharistic table. My question came in response to one friend who experienced the wine we were offering as a place of major temptation.

"He's participating in communion," my husband astutely said. "He knows what it is to drink from that cup of suffering *when he doesn't drink*. Help him reflect on that. Help him reflect on his participation in the cup of Jesus, on what he brings to the Cross, on where he is seeking new life and new creation."

We have a lens through which we view and understand and make meaning of the brokenness in which we live. This very real and very troubled relationship with food is not going away and can't be ignored. Our frayed and fractured relationship with food offers one more entry point into the blessed and broken road we walk with Jesus.

The Living Diet

Fasting

> O may our inmost hearts be pure,
> Our thoughts from folly kept secure,
> The pride of sinful flesh subdued
> By temperate use of daily food.[3]

✿ ✿ ✿

Our goal is . . . to become painfully aware, to dare to turn what is happening to the world into our own personal suffering and thus to discover what each of us can do about it.

—Pope Francis, *Laudato Si: On Care for our Common Home*[4]

---

3. "Hymns for Morning #4," *Common Praise* 1938, trans. 1851 from the Latin (5th century) by Rev. John M. Neale (Toronto: Anglican Book Centre, 1938), 3.

4. *Laudato Si, "On Care for our Common Home,"* Encyclical II from Pope Francis, June 18, 2015. *http://w2.vatican.va/content/francesco/en/encyclicals/documents/papa-francesco_20150524_enciclica-laudato-si.html.*

The Lenten Fast

As I said earlier, Lent is a forty-day season in the Christian calendar modeled on the forty days Jesus spent in the wilderness fasting before beginning his public ministry. Here are a few things to consider when embarking on the practice of an annual Lenten fast.

Food A few years ago, I gave up my favorite radio program for Lent. I had good spiritual reasons for doing so, but I decided that it let me off the hook with other things. The day after Ash Wednesday saw us at our neighbor's house for a fun family evening of fellowship and eating. Although Dan was doing a true Lenten fast, refraining from wine and any superfluous food consumption, I threw myself qualm-free into the meal. There were several other parties through Lent that I had also decided were okay for me to enjoy without restriction.

I was faithful in my chosen discipline, but I came to the end of Lent feeling that I had cheated. It wasn't some self-imposed guilt trip. Rather, I recognized the contrast between this Lent and previous Lenten fasts. I had missed out by not missing out. By not choosing a more restrained mode of eating, I had missed out on an important part of what Lent can be.

Christians have found many creative ways of observing Lent: giving up video games or television, offering more money to a particular charitable project, volunteering somewhere for the forty days. These can be effective and meaningful disciplines. But using Lent as a time for conscious choices about what we put into our bodies offers a particular opportunity for learning not afforded by any other versions of the fast.

Reasons. The risk in a Lenten fast involving food is that it can easily be coopted into the most destructive of Western cultural obsessions, dressed up as a spiritual search. I'm talking about weight loss. If a Lenten fast becomes one more diet attempt, one more yo on the yo-yo of loss and gain, then the discipline needs to be adjusted. Or at least the attitude to the discipline needs to be adjusted. Or at least it is worth observing, praying about, and learning from how seductive the cultural value of thinness is as it worms its way into our most tried and true spiritual practices.

Time. Whether you are religious or not, Lent is a good time to challenge yourself to be thoughtful about food and restraint. Ancient people knew something about time intuitively. The number forty recurs throughout scripture—forty days of the flood, forty years in the wilderness, forty days fasting. Forty was considered a powerful number spiritually, signifying a period of learning and spiritual growth. Forty days is the right amount of time. Furthermore, it is *at* the right time. The timing of Lent shifts according to the moon's cycle and the date for Easter. But Lent literally means spring. In southern Ontario anyway, this means that these forty days take place as winter is having its final hurrah and spring is just beginning to seriously wage battle with the cold and snow, to wake up the earth, and to show the first signs of life returning in the powerful cycle of the seasons.

Open Invitation. A friend, who grew up in the Christian faith but is no longer an active participant, said, "I have a Muslim friend who is ten years older than I am and she is about to go into the month of Ramadan. I have worked with her each year when she fasts for religious reasons. We have been friends for fourteen years and her religion never comes up except during this time when I can't help envying the spirituality she experiences."

Numerous times in my own work, I have seen people on the fringe of church life become intrigued by the invitation of Lent and engage in the discipline of fasting. Once it is extracted from the guilt with which Lent has sometimes been laden, once Lenten discipline becomes a choice again, it is an invitation for learning and growing. You cannot abstain from something for forty days without receiving meaningful insight about yourself and the world in which you live, without also discovering the true freedom that comes with choosing *not* to have something that we *can* have.

Fasting as Prayer

As I mentioned at the outset, monastics regularly assume a practice of fasting as part of their normal pattern of life. The monastic rule is simple and provides a wise and measured approach for any person looking to reorder their relationship with food:

1. Seek moderation—not too much, not too little.
2. Eat at designated times.
3. Eat food appropriate to the season and the area where you live.

Note the motive behind this pattern of eating. No monastic order names weight loss as the reason for moderation and restraint in relationship with food. Remember, our problem with food is not merely physical, but also spiritual. To adopt the monastic pattern of eating without also considering its spiritual foundations is to miss out on the big picture of health and wellness.

John Cassian, a monastic teacher, posits that our eating practices begin as thoughts. We can make choices about our thoughts; we bear responsibility for our thoughts. Monastic Mary Margaret Funk writes:

> When we feel the bodily need of food and drink, we begin to notice our thoughts about food and we know we must let them go without acting on them if we hope to progress in calming our mind. . . . If we can't tame the thought of food, there is no hope of getting control of the more difficult thoughts, such as sex and anger. The food thought is good in itself but can become an affliction when the thought compels the thinker into consent without discretion.[5]

When moderate fasting becomes a pattern of life, a recognition of abundance follows. Out of the abundance with which I have been blessed, I can share what I do not need with others. Moderation and abundance lead to a more just distribution of resources. There is enough. There is more than enough.[6]

Cooking for Allergies

We have a friend who is unable to eat wheat, dairy, soy, eggs, peanuts, or corn. Because wheat and corn are used in minute amounts in so many of our processed foods (so small in fact that companies are off

---

5. Funk, *Thoughts Matter*, 17.

6. Ibid., 18–23 outlines this basic pattern of possibilities that we can anticipate through adopting the fast of moderate eating.

the hook in terms of having to even include them on the labels), she can't eat most packaged foods, even something as simple as a can of diced tomatoes. She does not have life-threatening allergies, she assured me the first time we invited her to dinner. In fact, it took her years to discover that it was the food she was eating that was contributing to her feeling so miserable all the time because each allergy in and of itself was comparatively mild. The difference in her life between an unrestricted diet and the one that she now observes is night and day. When she follows the needs of her body, she can work and run a half marathon and play in her community band and go on canoe trips in the wilderness. When she doesn't, she can't get out of bed.

If you have done any exploration into your own relationship to different foods, you have probably discovered that there are things that your body has a harder time digesting—foods that weigh you down, bloat you out, make it hard to think, cause weight fluctuations, or induce indigestion. Or you might know what it is to suffer from an allergy that can kill you. You might have to be constantly prepared with an EpiPen® for the possibility of your body shutting down in response to a substance that others can enjoy as a healthy part of their diet.

You may believe that you can eat anything. You may have, like me, been schooled in the "everything in moderation" approach and may find the proliferation of allergies and intolerances confusing or even a little indulgent.

Because of the number of different eating difficulties that people face, because of the many individuals who are deciding that they are sick and tired of feeling sick and tired and are prepared to radically change their eating lifestyles, food has become a major source of division between people. Our friend will opt out of a restaurant dinner with others because of the stress of trying to find food she can eat. Other friends I know will bring their own food to potluck suppers because it is easier than having to eat things that will make them unwell.

The Living Diet invites you to choose communion over isolation. Make a point of sharing a meal with those who need restraint in order to be well. Talk to your friend or family member about their dietary regime, why they have had to give up certain foods, and what the difference has been in their lives. Allow their stories to resonate with the

questions implicit in what they are telling you: Why are these traditionally nutritious foods now causing harm to so many people? What are
we collectively doing to our food systems that has caused this reaction
to so many ancient food staples? Look for common ground. Look for
how "bread" can still be broken with one another. What restaurant will
accommodate the expressed needs? If you cook, what research can you
do, and what foods can you serve that will be enjoyable and life-giving
for all involved?

Close Call

Food is relationship. The difficulties so many of us have with consuming everyday foods is emblematic of the fractures that run across
our human relationships and between us and our earth. The effort we
make to eat together, in spite of these fractures, is a reaching across the
chasm, to choose communion over isolation, healing over brokenness.
Which is why these questions are so important: What are my eating
needs? What are my eating preferences? In other words, what do I have
to ask from others in order to be able to eat with them? What can I let
go of in order to bridge the gap?

As monastic Mary Margaret Funk reminds us, "To stay at the common table is a particular discipline."[7] Figuring out how to stay at the
table involves give and take from all of us, and a particular amount of
give and take from each of us according to our own understanding of
our body's needs. Asking the questions that lead us to the discipline of
staying at that common table, navigating together that cost, is perhaps
the most consequential part of the Living Diet.

Nail It to the Cross

I feel an almost physical repulsion toward any phrase that sounds
like a Christian cliché used by religious insiders. At one point in
my faith journey, Christianity had become so meaningless—or perhaps confusing—to me that basic statements like "Jesus is the Son of

---

7. Ibid., 28.

God" or "Jesus died for our sins" caused me to want to run out of the church screaming. It was only the fact that I was being paid to sing in the choir that kept me in my seat. Later on, when I was blessed enough to study with several superb theology professors, these overused statements began to mean something to me. Even so, I try to be careful about using them unless I am also going to say something about why they matter. So, I am a little hesitant to lay out this next possibility in the Living Diet: *nail it to the cross*.

It is a terribly clichéd Christian statement, too often offered as a quick response to human suffering, or sometimes as a humorous barb at someone who is being too melodramatic about their difficulties. Either way, it is based in the belief that because of Jesus's suffering, my own can better be borne, or even alleviated. For someone who is borderline religious or who is religious in a logical and intellectual sort of way, the statement might sound nothing short of ridiculous. And yet . . .

One year as Dan and I were moving through our Lenten fasts we began to discern that we were growing apart from a couple of dear friends. We both grieved at our realization. These people meant a great deal to us, but their lives were becoming more and more structured around the need to drink and we felt that we couldn't join them on that road. At one point in our sadness, the words slipped out of me. I had never said words like that before. I didn't know where they came from or how I meant them—*if* I meant them. I said them in a way that could have allowed me to claim them as ironic, depending on how Dan reacted. "Oh well, we have to nail it to the cross."

We both felt an immediate sense of relief from our sadness. It was an image that surprisingly meant something to us.

Our Christian faith is full of poetry and image. In contrast to all of the practices that we can *do* in the Living Diet, there are also practices in which we can simply dwell. Whether it is the cross, the broken bread of communion, the cup of suffering we claim as Jesus's blood, or the wounds on Jesus's hands and feet and side that convince the disciples after the Resurrection that Jesus is real and true, there is rich imagery in which we can locate our suffering in the bigger story of sacrifice and compassion.

The Living Diet will inevitably lead you to places where your food choices become choices for sacrifice. There will be foods that you will find that either permanently, or in certain company or at certain times, you will choose not to eat. You will choose not to eat because of the needs of others, because of the needs of the world, or because your body's own wellness has been implicated in the systems and structures of food production. You may fast from certain foods. You may very well experience these sacrifices as sadness. It could feel as if you are giving up a good friend or a part of your identity. You might believe that giving up a beloved food or drink is impossible. If you are going to take seriously this part of the Living Diet, if you are going to find within yourself the capacity to refrain from eating or drinking something that you *can* eat or drink, resources like prayer, symbol, and poetry may afford you a strength that mere willpower cannot. Consider these possibilities:

- **Surrender to a higher power:** The AA recovery program is famous for listing among its first steps the need to surrender to a higher power, however the individual chooses to define it. The ability to refrain from using a substance that I can use, and want to use, becomes not an act of willpower, but a recognition of how little power I have, an act of turning that power over to another.

- **Offer it up, nail it to the cross:** These are two of those clichéd religious phrases that can actually afford a powerful prayer image, a poetic visualization for the loss that we might encounter in our relationship with food. If you find it difficult to give up a food or a drink that you love, bring that sacrifice into this image, this poetry. Visualize your sacrifice as a thing that you can hold in your hand. See yourself giving that thing into the safekeeping of bigger, stronger hands. Or imagine that thing as a wisp of dandelion fluff, and as you lift your hands up, see that wisp carried out of your embrace and into the heavens. Let the cross, the nails, the wounded hands and feet, the blood, the suffering, act as poetry. Let your own experience slip into those graphic images, that they might represent some of the confusion and difficulty you are encountering. Let those words and images do the work of sacrifice for you, as good poetry has always done, expressing the depth of your difficulty and longing, carrying you through from a place of suffering to an experience of new life.

- **Go to church**: Whether you attend an Episcopal Eucharist, a Roman Catholic Mass, a Baptist "Lord's Supper," or whatever communion service you can find, you can do more than visualize and pray on your own. You can actually enact these symbols with a gathered group of people whose lives also contain fracture and sacrifice. You can hear that bigger story of suffering and resurrection, and you too can physically come forward, get on your knees, open your hands to receive, and have your life joined into the body of Christ. You don't have to believe the right things. You don't have to understand the mystery. Just allow yourself to participate with others in acting out in our bodies our own surrender, our own offering-up and taking-in.

chapter

15

Run for Life

started running to lose weight. I *became* a runner by accident.

I was the kid who was always picked last for teams in gym class. I dreaded team sports, gymnastics, anything requiring agility and coordination. But I especially dreaded the days when we had to run. While everyone else was able to show their prowess on the track without much obvious effort, I huffed and puffed from the get-go, sure that my lungs and legs were on the verge of giving out. In grade 8, we had to run laps every week around our little gymnasium, counting how many we could do in a certain amount of time and then reporting our number to our teacher. Out loud. In front of the entire class. I was so humiliated by my dead-last number that honesty went by the wayside, and I started occasionally miscounting. (I don't feel as badly about this now when I pause to wonder why the teacher never taught us anything about the form or technique that would have allowed us to honestly improve.) I was still last.

It was a happy day when I finished grade 9 gym. After that, phys ed was no longer a required course. Knowing I could pursue the rest of my career as a student without the daily dread of embarrassment and exhaustion and incompetence hanging over me was like being given a winning lottery ticket.

Athletics did hold one appeal for me though. When my friends chose some kind of sport as the "fun" activity of the day—tennis, swimming, skiing, soccer—I suffered through the ordeal by daydreaming.

What would my body look like if *this time* I discovered there was a latent athlete within me? I imagined playing a sport and being so naturally good at it that I suddenly became sporty and fit. My body, of course, played a central role in my daydream. My body became fit and sporty and thin in the process. That dream never amounted to anything. I never discovered a hidden athletic talent. I only felt a vast sense of relief when the sport of the day was over and I could stop embarrassing myself and return to more sedentary pursuits.

When I began university, family members and upper-year classmates warned ominously about "The Frosh 15" weight gain. I managed to eat fairly balanced meals; my parents had instilled reasonably good habits in me. But it was the late-night lifestyle that caught up with all of us. Even the skinniest girl on my floor, the scarecrow-thin Erin, began to complain about her small stomach pouch. We tried to avoid beer and the most sugary alcoholic drinks and stuck to diet-pop mixers. But it was still too many extra calories. And those calories led to other calories. When you've had a few drinks and you've been out dancing all night and it's been a long time since you had supper, you don't have any steel to guard yourself against the host of late-night food options: pizza, potato chips, poutine. In London, Ontario, we had Sammy's Souvlaki, a food cart conveniently positioned outside of the most popular bars, and we feasted on falafels and gyros wrapped in warm flatbreads and dripping with oils and sauces as we figured out how to get home.

"Well, we're not going to stop drinking," Erin said, in a voice as thin as she was, "and we can't get fat. So we're going to have to do something."

Our university was well-equipped with exercise facilities, so we trudged up the hill for aerobics classes. We felt great after the first class. "I'm not even that hungry," my friend May commented. We had found the solution. We each attended about three classes the entire year. Weight loss seemed like a great motivator, but when it came down to it, there was almost always something better to do than go and sweat to somebody else's workout.

That first year did, however, open the door for me to begin dabbling in an erratic smattering of exercise endeavors. When I came home that summer, about ten pounds heavier—not too bad, considering—I began jogging a bit with my dad. The weight came off quickly and so I kept up the practice periodically through the summer. I would picture the skinny body I wanted to have and try to motivate myself to continue on. It was only a moderately successful incentive.

In my third year, we planned a trip to Florida for spring break. I desperately wanted to be able to wear a bikini. I took up a regular fitness regime of one half hour on the bike machine a few times a week. That, in combination with the "herbal" diet pills I began taking, worked wonders. I put all the weight back on by the time we came home from Florida.

In year four, I took the promising advice of a different friend and began weightlifting. "That's the secret," Jessica told me enthusiastically. "You build muscle, and the fat just melts away. When I was weight lifting, I had the most incredible back. I would get comments from strangers about how good my back looked." She had named my dangling carrot: me in a slinky backless top. My boyfriend and I began daily two-hour weight-lifting sessions at the university gym. No fat melted away, but my appetite certainly increased, and I ended my undergrad career at my heaviest.

I continued with my half-hearted exercise efforts—half-hearted because they were always a means toward the one unreachable end of shedding pounds. I ran sometimes. I lifted weights for a while. I got on the StairMaster occasionally. I had an old bicycle that I began using for transportation when I was working in Oakville. I knew nothing about maintaining it and rode around on flat tires for months before my colleague Michael told me I should probably look at investing in a tire pump. Although I was in a healthier relationship with my body by then, I fleetingly wondered if I would burn as many calories riding on inflated tires.

Occasionally I would leave my bike at the office and then run to work the next day. It was seven kilometers from my apartment to the church where I worked. I would run part of the way, walk part of the way, and then bike home. It was great exercise, but more importantly, it diminished my carbon footprint and was easier on my lean financial resources, and so, as my schedule allowed, this became my commuting habit of choice.

It was on one of these runs that I first experienced what it is for the rhythm of the running to lull me into self-forgetfulness. I stopped worrying about how I was getting cramps in my side and how my lungs were parched for air. That anxious voice inside asking, "how much longer?" was temporarily quiet.

When I starting thinking and processing again, I realized that I felt great. Running felt great. There was an almost musical cadence to my stride. My breathing was light and easy. A strange sense of exhilaration coursed through my veins. I began talking with other runners, comparing notes on my discovery. It was adrenaline, not weight loss, that finally led me to describe myself as a runner. Gradually that time on my feet became not a chore, not a dieting device, but a valued part of my life.

Years later, after ups and downs with knee problems, the births of two children, the discovery of the need for diligence in picking out, caring for, and regularly replacing running shoes, I was talking to my friend Jeff, a superhero marathon runner type, who reflected, "The people who are good at running, who are actually competitive and win races, they are people who have found joy."

His words have proven to be true. I don't have to win races. But I rejoice in my own improvements, I set goals for myself, and running is now one of the single most important activities in my life. It is my time for prayer, reflection, problem-solving, imagining, and noticing connections and patterns in my own experience of the world around me. I try to remember, at the beginning of each run, to give thanks to God for giving me a body that can be on the move, that can get me from one destination to another at just the right pace to see and feel the road I'm on, that can reward me with a buzzing sense of wellness for the effort that feels like it is never solely my own.

It's not a joke to say that I am the poster girl for the claim that everyone can run. I love to talk about running because I can do so without bragging. I am not athletic. I am the ultimate clumsy and nerdy book worm. It was no great act of determination and discipline that led me to become a runner. I am the most unlikely candidate for adopting a regular discipline of running, let alone enjoying it. Running isn't something that I chose; it chose me.

A Damaging Lifestyle

A study released in 2013 found a link between the decline in the number of hours women were spending doing housework and the rise of female obesity.[1] It was the kind of headline clearly meant to grab attention and stir the pot of controversy. You can just imagine the outrage and the punch lines in response. But the study is really nothing more than a rehashing of what we already know. It is the complement to another study that tracked changes in physical activity in the workplace. Jobs have become more sedentary for both men and women. Their conclusions point to the same things we have been noting for years as our culture tries to come to terms with our waistlines. We are spending more time than ever—whether for leisure or for work—*sitting* in front of screens.

Lead researcher Edward Archer wisely concluded his study by stating that more housework for women is not the answer to the problem. I say "wisely" because I doubt he wanted to be at the butt end of the feminist rage that such a suggestion would raise. I find some humor in picturing women (and men) across the continent starting the new Housework Program, equipping themselves with mops and buckets and committing to forty-five minutes of floor cleaning three times a week. (Is there any more horrible thought?) I can also imagine that Housework Program mop and bucket eventually finding itself stacked on top of the unused treadmill, right next to the exercise ball and Beachbody DVDs.

Any study that notes a relationship between lack of movement and increased weight has to fall into the category of *Not Rocket Science*. I am much more interested in emerging research that looks at more than just weight when considering our health. A Chinese study released in 2014 covering hundreds of thousands of participants across several continents linked a sedentary lifestyle with a 25 percent increase in the incidence of depression.[2] Our physical health is linked to our spiritual

---

1. Jason Rehel, "It Sounds Sexist, but Women Doing Less Housework than in the 1960s May Be Related to the Obesity Epidemic: Study," *National Post*, February 28, 2013, *https://nationalpost .com/health/it-sounds-sexist-but-women-doing-less-housework-may-be-related-to-the-obesity-epidemic*.

2. Shereen Lehman, "Sedentary Lifestyle Linked to Depression," Reuters, September 18, 2014, *http:// www.reuters.com/article/2014/09/18/us-health-depression-sedentary-idUSKBN0HD2K120140918*.

and emotional health. Whether we look at housework in the home or manual labor in the workplace, our lifestyles are becoming less and less active and we miss the forest for the trees when we narrow in on one problem area—our waistlines—and ignore the bigger picture of damage we are inflicting on ourselves.

Consider any one of the thousands of commuters who make the daily multihour trek into Toronto from our small city of St. Catharines. A typical workday involves getting up at 4:45 a.m. to leave the house by 5:15 a.m. If the weather cooperates and there are no accidents on the highway, they can get ahead of the morning rush to catch the train on time. The train stops in the southern end of the city, close to the lake, so they also need subways, street cars, or city buses (or all three!) to get to work. At the end of the day, the commuter does the entire two-hour-plus commute again in reverse. They are perpetually exhausted. They want to build physical activity into their routine, but all spare time is taken up with commuting.

Because of my husband's particular fields of interest, Dan once ended up working in three churches, two universities, and a monastery (all at the same time) with his primary work being the completion of his doctoral thesis at his computer in our basement. Dan herniated a disc twice as he typed, sending him into mind-numbing pain and weeks of physiotherapy. When asked how he injured himself, he sheepishly had to admit, "Desk work."

In one episode of *The Office*, Michael Scott, the manager of a small paper supply company, tried to convince the warehouse workers that desk jobs were dangerous too. He spent a day demonstrating the risks associated with a sedentary lifestyle, culminating with orchestrating a mock suicide attempt from the roof of the office building. Nobody walked away from his efforts believing office work to be particularly dangerous, and yet the irony of this particular episode was that, of course, he was right. The depression and the physical damage that comes from sitting and staring into artificial light all day *is* dangerous. "Sitting is the new smoking" goes one slogan.

There are any number of products aimed at addressing this danger. Walking desks allow a treadmill to be attached to the standing work station. "Smart" watches buzz when we've been sitting too long, encouraging us to stand and stretch. Bigger companies have small gyms that employees are encouraged to use on breaks. Others businesses subsidize gym memberships. Without dismissing any of these solutions, the Living Diet offers a different perspective on building movement into our daily lives, and most importantly, for rethinking how and why we would choose to move more.

The Living Diet

Moving

Maybe buying that gym membership isn't going to be the best way to get active after all. This part of the Living Diet gives you strategies for thinking differently in order to move more.

Daily Commute

I am a full-time working mother. I sympathize with all of the reasons why we get out of shape. Every moment of my life is accounted for. At the end of the night, when the workday is done and the kids are in bed and the lunches are made for the next day and the kitchen is clean (sort of), the last thing that I want to do is put on my jogging shoes and go running. Motivation at that time of the day stretches no further than the fridge or the couch. But most of us have some time built into our day that we can use differently. We commute. Consider these options:

1. Ride your bike to work. If you live close enough, this is the easiest and most rewarding way of reclaiming some of your day. If you're not close enough to bike, it might still be an option. When I was working in Oakville and living in Hamilton (30 kilometers away, a little further than I felt I had time and energy for regularly biking), I arranged to leave my bike at a friend's garage halfway in between. I drove to her place and then biked the second fifteen kilometers to work. It actually saved me time; her house was at the same point on the commute where traffic became heavy and the maddening stop-and-go travelling began. At a later point in my life when I was living

twenty-five kilometers north of Oakville in Georgetown, I set biking the hilly back route to work as a summer goal, eventually accomplishing not only the mostly downhill trip there, but also the mostly uphill trip home. I didn't do it every day, but worked it in once or twice a week. As with most bike riding in busy city life, doing so didn't cost me much more time, but I did have to make sure that I packed enough food to fuel my way home.

2. Run to work. This option takes a little more planning, but is doable. It involves bringing an extra change of clothes, an extra lunch (if you're a brown bag lunch type), and your gym bag of running gear. At the end of the day, change into your running clothes and leave everything else at work. Don't forget your keys. Run home that evening and run back the next morning. Make sure to leave a stick of deodorant in your desk or with your change of clothes. After you get to work and allow a few minutes for the sweat to dry, change into clean clothes and freshen up.

3. Your commute may be farther than you can run; however, this plan might still work for a portion of the trip. The idea is that it doesn't require the finding of any more time in the day. Run instead of riding and you have gained energy, a mood boost, and a few more dollars in your pocket.

4. Walk to work. Walking is another way to commute and requires less planning than running. You can wear your work clothes. You can take your lunch with you in a backpack. You probably won't need a refresher of deodorant, but carrying an extra stick with you isn't a bad idea anyway. If you live in walking distance to work, that's great. If not, as above, pick a portion of the trip to briskly hoof it.

Second Uniform

As a parish priest, I often joke that my congregation never sees me in real clothes. On Sunday mornings, I wear a robe in worship. During the week when I'm leading meetings, I am inevitably in jogging pants. Rather than my casual wear signaling a lack of seriousness on my part, I believe instead that it increases my authority. I am communicating through my clothing that I choose to make my emotional and physical health—and therefore also spiritual health—a priority in my life. On a practical level, wearing my runners to an evening meeting makes it much more likely that, at the end of the meeting, I will actually run home, rather than tiredly opt out because even the thought of having to now get myself changed is one hurdle more than I can manage. My clothes signal that I am committed. My clothes make me accountable to the people around me who now also believe I am committed to run.

If you are in a position where you can set the rules about appropriate dress, and better yet, if you can articulate what those clothes mean about the choices you are making, consider using your power for the good of us all. Wouldn't it be wonderful if we lived in a world where a cotton running top was considered just as much a sign of professionalism as a power suit?

Become an Environmentalist

I often struggle with motivation. I have a life that leaves me feeling tired at the end of the day, and sometimes at points in between. I do not always feel like biking or jogging or going through the extra planning that either discipline requires. My motivation is rekindled, though, by any of the regular reminders that our planet is in great peril. They help me to remember that my choices are not just about me. If there is some small alternative that I can take—even occasionally—to pump fewer fossil fuels into the atmosphere, to leave a lighter footprint on the earth, then I can feel good about that, even as the convenience of the car tempts me otherwise.

Get Cheap

Frugality can be a good motivator. If you work out the average cost per mile in using your car, then it can be exciting to calculate how much money you save every time you choose an alternative. You can designate the saved money for something particular: a treat that you want or a nonprofit organization of your choice. Our kids' school set up an extended charity fundraiser, inviting friends and acquaintances to pledge a certain amount of money to new playground equipment for the miles that each teacher committed to making on bike or on foot through the year. Doing so also encouraged others—including the students—to think differently about their commute.

Parking

Back in the 1990s, when Sharon Stone was considered the hottest actress in Hollywood, I heard her interviewed about the secret to her fabulous body. "Oh," she said, "When I have to get ready for a particular role, I just begin to make some adjustments to my routine. You know, things like parking farther away when I go shopping." Her answer irritated me in the same way that my friends irritated me when one of them lost weight and then feigned nonchalance. I did not believe for a second that Sharon Stone got *Basic Instinct*–ready by walking a little further from the parking lot to her favorite outlet mall.

Nonetheless, I do recommend parking at the outside edge of the lot. The difference between the designated parking spot I used to have right next to the church building and the place I now park, on the edge of the lower lot, is 120 steps. I easily go from and to my car twice a day, which adds up to 480 steps. Five days a week, that is an extra 2,400 steps, which is almost two kilometers.

Getting into the habit of parking in the first available spot, rather than driving around to find a spot that is close, adds up to more walking for you and less fuel consumption for your car. If you walked just an extra 100 meters ten times a week—at work, at the grocery store, at the commuter train—that is an extra kilometer of walking that week *and* a kilometer less of driving. It is also more than just a kilometer of saved fossil fuels because stopping and starting and idling around a parking lot uses much more gas than is suggested by reading the odometer.

There is a caveat: park far from the door *only* if doing so means that you are driving less. In other words, don't drive around putting extra miles on your car simply so that you get more walking in. It's not just about you.

Jar of Marbles

There is a popular spiritual teaching tool that can be done with marbles. An empty peanut butter jar can be filled with marbles: one boulder, a bunch of small ones. However, they only all fit if you put them in the right order. If you put the small ones in first, the big one won't fit on the top. If you put the boulder in first though, all of the other ones fit around it.

It's used for teaching the importance of putting God in our lives first so that everything else fits. But it also reflects the counterintuitive dynamic of making room—one creative way or other—for physical activity in your life. Not surprisingly, it's about relationship. It is impossible to be emotionally and mentally well, not to mention spiritually, if you are ignoring your physical wellness. Weave exercise into your routine and discover that you also have time and energy for work, for family, for thinking clearly, for noticing the effects of prayer, for sleeping well, for relaxing with friends, for giving back to your community.

The First Ten Minutes Are the Worst

I discovered this truth while running, although it has applications in any realm of physical exercise, as well as in many other aspects of life: prayer, church worship, piano practice, meditation, lawn cutting. I have yet to test whether or not it works for vacuuming. In the first ten minutes, you will feel crampy and your breathing will be labored and your mind will cook up every possible alternative for what you could be doing. If you can get past the first ten minutes, that monkey on your shoulder will start to get bored, your breathing will find a rhythm, and adrenaline will get your muscles moving. In other words, your brain will let go of the need to analyze and reject your activity and will start to work holistically with the rest of your body. If you know the first ten minutes are the worst, you also know that it is worth it to push through to joy.

Prayer

The act of giving thanks for something changes your relationship to it. When you're moving, give thanks for what you are doing, for being *able* to do what you are doing. Pray about your physical activity as if it were a blessing and then discover how it starts to feel like one. While you're at it, consider adopting a simple prayer or meditative refrain while you're biking, running, or exercising. It can be an effective means of helping your body to find its rhythm. It is also an excellent reminder of how physical health is never merely about a physical outcome, but how our bodies are inwardly formed as relational. Exercise doesn't just affect your waist: it affects your mind, your emotions, your spirit, your soul.

Language

Melissa Etheridge had a song on the radio a few years ago about battling breast cancer called "Run for Life," and it has been the theme song for one of the biggest breast cancer fundraising runs. She names the women in her life for whom she runs, and then gathers all of these special relationships into the conclusion that why she really runs is "for life."

Though the poetry is simple and the melody is a little campy, the song chokes me up. My son, listening from the back seat of the car a few years ago, had a different take on it. "Why's she running for her life?" he asked. "Who's chasing her?" Knowing Gordon, he pictured the poor woman trying to escape a band of renegade pirates or something similarly adventurous.

The song's sentiment can be extended beyond a reflection on breast cancer. It is powerful to think of the exercise we do as serving purposes much bigger than just weight loss and waistlines. It is powerful to claim exercise as something other than a dirty job we have to do in order to look a certain way. It is powerful to think that the activity in which we engage is part of our service to our families and to the world around us. It is powerful because it allows physical activity to take its rightful place in our lives, not as one more discipline to adopt, but as part and parcel of a meaningful, other-centered life.

16

Body Language

> Most of my students can't imagine a world in which they would stop
> dieting or trying to fix the size of their thighs. It is easier to imagine
> people coming back from the dead or Brad Pitt asking them to get
> married than to imagine themselves dropping the war with their
> bodies. They have whole friendships built on commiserating about
> the twenty pounds they have to lose and the jeans that are too tight
> and the latest greatest diets. They fit in by hating themselves.
>
> —Geneen Roth, *Women, Food & God*

What's in a Name?

Anne Shirley, famous red-headed orphan from the book *Anne of Green Gables*, arrived at her new home spouting a steady stream of chatter as she reflected on the mysteries of the world around her and the deepest questions of her hungry soul. "I read somewhere," she said, "that a rose by any other name would still smell as sweet, but I just can't believe it. I just don't think that it would be the same if it were called a thistle or a skunk-cabbage!"

Anne's insistence that her name be spelled with an "e" because "Anne" was an entirely different name than "Ann" touches on a long-held truth in the significance of names. Spiritually speaking, names are important. In the biblical Creation story, Adam reveals something of what it means to be "created in the image and likeness of God" by naming the creatures that God made. Adam took part in God's creative work. The witness of scripture confirms that humankind has had a hand in shaping the world around us because to name is to essentially decide something about what those things will be, their qualities and characteristics.

This power of naming is assumed throughout the pages of the Bible. When God called Abram and Sarai to participate in the divine covenant, to be the first generation to walk with God in a newly intimate way and therefore reveal God's faithfulness to all people, God recognized their choice and chosenness by renaming them. They become Abraham, which means "father of many nations," and Sarah, which means "princess" or "noblewoman."

Jesus was named by his father, Joseph, directed by angelic instruction. His name means "God saves." Later in Jesus's life, when he was beginning to call his disciples, he insisted on one of the most famous name changes since his ancestors Abraham and Sarah. Simon was renamed *Petros*: Peter, or "The Rock." There was nothing obviously rocklike about fisherman Simon, Son of John. He was a man of fleeting passions, who plunged headfirst into the intuitive darkness of faith, but was also easily swayed by his fear and ego. He was the first to identify Jesus as the Messiah, and also the first to misunderstand that Jesus's messiahship did not mean a first-class ticket to earthly power and glory. He attempted to correct his teacher when Jesus predicted that his road led to suffering and death, then joined the disciples in nattering with one another through most of the rest of Jesus's ministry. He made heroic claims around the supper table prior to Jesus's arrest ("though all become deserters because of you, I will never desert you"), only to deny knowing Jesus—three times, no less—a few hours later.

Simon was not a rock. He was bendable, permeable, shifting, soft. And yet, quietly and persistently, the power of his new name emerged. "You are Peter, and on this rock I will build my church." Despite all of his malleability and cloudiness, Peter came back to his Lord. Peter received forgiveness. Peter was commissioned as a shepherd of the sheep. And after Jesus's resurrection appearances, Peter became a key leader in the early church, identified by many as "first among the apostles."

The name "Peter" helped to shape who he became.

Dan and I marvel at how well our children's names fit them. Cecilia, named partly for St. Cecilia the patron saint of music, has been matching pitch since she was a baby and composing songs since she was two years old. Gordon, named after my grandfather, shares much of my grandfather's kind and generous personality, his wicked sense of humor, and his big caring heart. Likewise, I have come to identify strongly with the biblical character Martha. Above my desk are printed Jesus's words to his friend on the night that he ate with her and her sister, Mary: "Martha, Martha, you are worried and distracted by many things; there is need of only one thing" (Luke 10:41–42). I get caught up in the tasks of life, and like Martha, occasionally need to be reminded of the gracious witness of Mary, who made time to sit and listen at Jesus's feet.

Even thousands of years after these biblical witnesses, we still experience the power of names. The names we give and the ways that we choose to speak about one another do more than identify us; they actually shape who we and the world around us are becoming.

Body Talk

I used to fantasize about pregnancy as a time when I could get fat and enjoy it. I could eat whatever I wanted without worrying about my hips and tummy. Instead, when I actually did begin to show with my first child, I was shocked at the fat language that got thrown around. "Fat" no longer seemed like an appropriate word to describe the incredible thing my body, without any instruction, knew how to do.

"Oh, you're in your fat pants now," someone in my congregation commented to me when I first broke out the maternity wear.

"Hold your stomach in," another parishioner reminded me. I was resentful about those comments for weeks. Only much later did I realize that the obvious absurdity of telling a pregnant woman to hold in her stomach might have offered insight into the assumptions and insecurities of the person making the comment but was certainly not valid advice for me in how to carry my growing baby bump.

These comments were offensive, but atypical. The more routine remarks were from people asking me how much weight I had put on and then passing judgment about whether or not that was appropriate.

"Good for you," some would say. "It's all baby. You're doing well." Others felt compelled to share their own memories: "I only put on fifteen pounds in my whole pregnancy." These anecdotes were not help-ful, nor was I convinced that they hadn't been falsified by time and our human penchant for exaggerating our storytelling. I started to feel an unexpected kinship with movie stars. Somehow celebrities and pregnant women invite a sense of entitlement in others to publicly scrutinize their weight. Our ravenous interest in the added pounds of others says far more about our disordered view of the human body than it does about Britney Spears or a woman with a gloriously round baby belly.

The scrutiny became so severe that I had to do something. I was entering my third trimester just as Lent was beginning. As I discussed in chapter 6, men and women often give up a particular luxury for the sake of others during Lent. Any Lenten discipline is meant as a means of drawing closer to God—letting go of clutter, making room for what is real and true.

I had already given up a great deal in order to be pregnant. Preg-nancy is its own fast. I wasn't drinking. My caffeine consumption was limited. I had had to cut back on some activities because my body was diverting my energy to this priority of creating new life. I reflected on my experience with my spiritual director Audrey and decided that the most appropriate discipline for me that year was taking up simple acts that would remind me of the beauty of my own body.

I committed to having a sweet-smelling bubble bath once a week. I rubbed a rich body butter on my growing stomach each night before bed, enjoying the feel of the lotion seeping into my taut skin. I painted my toes and tried not to bite my finger nails.

That might sound frivolous or self-centered. It wasn't expensive. I didn't use my discipline as an excuse for buying a bunch of meaningless products or treating myself to shopping extravaganzas. As simple as it sounds, it changed my attitude. It changed the way I reacted to the silly comments of others. It neutralized my anger and frustration. There was a newfound firmness in my voice when I said, "Oh, let's not talk about pregnancy that way." My insistence on speaking properly about what was happening to me and my promise to feel beautiful in the expe-rience impacted me, and I hope that in a small way it impacted the people around me. What we say and feel about our own bodies sends powerful messages to others.

Children

> If any of you put a stumbling block before one of these little ones
> who believe in me, it would be better for you if a great millstone
> were fastened around your neck and you were drowned in the
> depth of the sea. (Matt. 18:6)

I gave birth to a daughter. Two years later, I had a son. Parenthood triggered a deep sense of responsibility in me. Cecilia will grow up with one (very thin) female body type represented in all of the vast variety of media she will consume through YouTube, films, television, cartoons, magazines, even dolls. Her girlfriends will obsess about their weight and body development, perhaps as early as grade 4 or 5. If she takes after me, she will struggle with athletics. Gordon will face his own body pressures. Our increasing awareness of male body image difficulties and male eating disorders could mean that we are becoming better able to identify and respond to body troubles in our young men. Or it could be an indication that the pressures for young men are increasing. Both of my children will be exposed to, and will eventually be at liberty to buy, any number of unhealthy diet options, from pop laced with aspartame, to unbalanced fad diets, to weight loss shakes, to diet pills, steroids, and "herbal remedies."

I was raised in a home of love and acceptance. My mother was the guiding light who led me through my difficult preadolescent years when I was taunted relentlessly by the other girls in my class. I was lost, awkward, and alone. My mother never once chided me about my weight or made me feel that I was anything less than acceptable the way that I was. My parents together made an unwavering commitment to serving balanced, healthy meals in our house. And they taught me that indulging together in a special dessert was a treat to enjoy, not an interior battle of willpower where restraint and appetite locked horns.

I picked up some other messages too, though. I learned from the world around me that stomachs looked best flat. I learned that dieting was a normal and acceptable part of life. I came to believe, as early as grade 4, that I should be dieting.

Cecilia and Gordon will be exposed to a terrifying number of subtle, insipid, and homogenous messages about what sort of body each should have. I understand that I bear an enormous responsibility to at least counter those messages on the home front, which takes a conscious effort. It is easy to slip into lifelong learned behavior around how I talk about my body. If I am not paying attention, I find myself pushing the right behaviors in the wrong way; with the best of intentions I can end up modelling destructive attitudes and practices.

After I had Cecilia and then Gordon, I began praying in thanksgiving, particularly in the long hours I spent with each of them breastfeeding. I found myself marveling at the wonders my body had participated in, for the babies that grew in my uterus, that were shuttled into the world through my body and fed by my milk—all miraculous occurrences of my body having the intuitive ability to create and form and deliver and feed a brand new life. I decided I wanted to carry that prayer forward, even when they each in turn stopped nursing. Now running seems the most appropriate time to offer that gratitude. I feel the joy that comes from my muscles and bones and lungs and heart and blood all working together, and I make a point of saying a word of thanks to God.

Out of that prayer, I have developed some guidelines for "body language"—how I seek to speak about my body. Like exercise and training, this regular discipline allows me to find my balance even when I find myself occasionally slipping on the banana peels of life.

The Living Diet

Speaking

We are culturally a long way off from reclaiming healthy attitudes toward our bodies. We can, however, change our attitudes by first changing our language. Our words and our names are powerful. This power can be destructive. It can be an uphill climb to break patterns, to live into a different reality than the ones we have been named into. And this power can be life-giving, shaping us into the people we were always meant to be, living in a world teaming with God's blessings.

The following language tips can be adopted without necessarily first believing what is being said. The names we choose to give

Continued

The Living Diet *Continued*

ourselves and the world around us begin to influence how we, and how our world, will actually be. Think back to the experiment with the water crystals, the microscopic change in their appearance, depending on which words have been spoken over them. The words that we choose to verbalize and the names that we express out loud do begin not just to change our own perception of a thing, but the thing itself. To say my body is beautiful is not just, in other words, to help me *see* that my body is beautiful, it is to *make* my body more beautiful as well.

Don't use phrases like "I feel fat" or "I need to lose weight." If, medically, you actually do need to lose weight, talk about weight loss in the context of what is necessary for your health.

Don't trash your body in front of other people. I have a hazy memory, from my early twenties, of getting ready to go out with friends for a night of dancing. As usual, I was feeling upset about my body. Two of us were last to leave. The girl that I was with was a friend of a friend, not someone I knew well. And she was overweight. I could see that she had some mild breathing and mobility issues as a result. And yet, without a thought to how my words would impact her, I primped in front of the mirror, sucked in my stomach, and whined, "Oh, I feel so fat!"

"I don't know how you can say that," she said quietly. I came out of my own self-absorption long enough to see the crestfallen look on her face. *If she thinks she looks fat, what must she think about me?*

If you have trouble with how you are physically or emotionally feeling about how you look, work that out in private. Remember that how we talk about our bodies in public can affect how others deal with their relationship to their bodies. Remember, too, that negative words spoken about your body can do physical harm to your body's ability to serve your needs; exist in a holistic partnership with your entire being.

Don't link your dietary choices with weight loss. My wise friend Gloria, a nutritionist and alternative-health care proponent, helps a lot of people lose weight. She never promises to help people lose weight. She promises to help them feel better. Push back against the relentless weight loss obsessions. If you can speak of your food choices based on the energy you need, the strength you are able to build, the improvements to your digestion and mental well-being, or even better, about how your choices can impact positively on the world around you, you can be part of carving out little pockets of space where all of us can create a different relationship with our bodies.

Ditch phrases like "That brownie went right to my hips" and "I just look at those potato chips and I put on five pounds." If you indulge, savor it, be grateful for it. This takes practice.

Speak about how your body *feels*, not how it looks. If you indulged and it was a mistake—it was mindless or destructive—center your reaction on the experience of your body. For example, I don't sleep well after having chocolate in the evening. My husband experiences sinus congestion and extreme fatigue after eating a doughnut. Both of us can speak of our need to make different choices based on the signals our bodies are sending us.

Make a habit of speaking of the other signals your body sends you. Many of us become disconnected from our bodies' most basic signals about hunger and fullness. Notice when you are full and then stop eating. Notice when you are hungry and eat.

Treat your body like your best friend. Perhaps the lines of communication with your friend have become strained or lazy in recent years. Commit to habits that allow those lines to open up again, to heal. Become an advocate for your body; speak of it in good and grateful terms. Your body is the one friend you actually *have* to live with!

Bring prayer into your relationship with your body. Take a moment to pray for peace in our world and to give thanks for the things that your body allows you to do. Give thanks for your food before you consume it. Even better, take a moment after you eat to feel—not guilt, not regret, not dissatisfaction—but celebration and gratitude for what you have been able to receive.

Bring joy into your language. Practice speaking to others about the joy of eating, and the related joys of buying and preparing food. You will, no doubt, surprise people. Our culture predominantly sees cooking as a chore, grocery shopping as a waste of time and money, and eating as an act that is best celebrated by the ways in which we are able to restrain ourselves. I used to feel that I had to hide how much I ate, or how much I wanted to eat. Over time I have learned to include food in any description of what brings me joy in life.

Disconnect exercise from weight loss. Don't link exercise to weight loss or compensation for guilt over eating the wrong things. Discover the capacity to enjoy physical activity for the way it makes you feel. Let your decision to exercise be about the choice to feel good, not to "burn off last night's dessert." Note, too, that physical health allows you to better fulfill other responsibilities you have in your life, and not only that, but your choices for running, walking, or biking to the store have a positive impact on more than just you.

Do you hate to exercise? Believe me, I was the queen of hating exercise (see some of the notes and experiences of the previous chapter). But I will again say that if you even begin by making a choice to speak differently about exercise, I promise that this change in words will eventually change the way that you feel.

These are some of the body language guidelines for how you speak about yourself, but there are a few important guidelines for speaking to others too:

Don't ever fall into the trap of greeting others with the classic, "You look great—have you lost weight?" I can't even begin to count how many times I have seen people at their most unhealthy—consumed with worries for their health, facing cancer scares or even in the middle of treatment, in and out of doctors' appointments and waiting to see specialists, or battling eating disorders—and because they have lost weight are bombarded with comments about how great they look. Thin does not equal wellness, and tying these two things to one another can be destructive and demoralizing. If you want to be complimentary about how someone looks, leave weight out of it.

If you are a parent, link your eating guidelines for your children to the signals their bodies send them. Cecilia becomes grouchy and overly sensitive when she has eaten too much sugar. Gordon's stomach hurts when he eats dairy. Rather than speaking of calories or fat, I try to help them identify how they feel after they have over-indulged. As they get older, I will help them to notice when their language about their bodies is disrespectful.

Be prepared for people to mishear you. I once wrote a piece on my blog about the controversy surrounding a Canadian celebrity who was under fire for alleged sexual assault. My goal was to name the various voices I was hearing in the culture, as well as the sequence of my own mixed emotions. It was not a perfectly expressed piece of writing, and it raised intense online ire from people particularly sensitive to our collective tendency to "blame the victim" and to unwittingly promote rape culture. One of the things for which I was attacked was my call to forgiveness toward this fallen icon. I can appreciate the perspective. Who am I to decide that someone who has been hurt should forgive their aggressor? Except I had never suggested that forgiveness was what was needed. I had never used the word "forgiveness" in that particular writing at all. Because the conversation going on in the culture around my writing was rife with musings on forgiveness, my critics had read it onto my writing as well.

We hear what we think we're hearing. We read the words that we expect. I talk about food a lot. I talk about how much I enjoy eating and how some foods make me feel bad. I never talk about needing to lose weight or how many calories I have just consumed. But I know that sometimes people hear in my very carefully chosen words the other messages that they are used to hearing. These inevitable breakdowns in communication are good reminders of how important a shift in language actually is, how far we have to still go in our language to reshape our relationship to food and bodies.

The need to choose my words well took on particular urgency when I had children. Because I try not to speak about wanting or needing to lose weight, I notice how much others do talk about that. I like bucking the trend and not joining in with my own dieting woes. I like the message that I send when I speak of how much I love food and love eating, not only to my children, but also to friends and acquaintances, and when I *don't* follow those sentiments with a lament for the havoc it wreaks on my figure.

My husband would no doubt say that I am a pest when it comes to his eating habits, but I try to make it clear, to him and to our kids, that my concern is for his health, not his appearance. I have worked hard to model better body image behavior. I haven't quite scaled the mountainous challenge of balancing my wish for my husband's health with my need to be supportive and loving.

I slip occasionally. If I am tired or strung-out or feeling low, that "f" word can still escape my lips. *Fat.* Clichés like "practice makes perfect" and "if at first you don't succeed, try, try again," might be overused, but they do speak truth. I also bank on the prayer of Jesus which suggests that in my own willingness to forgive the shortcomings of others, God will bless me with a gentle mercy. My feeble and flawed attempts to change my language do build muscles that give me strength against all of the food and body pitfalls that surround me. And I pray that they have some positive impact on the people around me too.

What Do We Want?
Everything!

A house doctor on a public broadcasting morning talk show listed things he wished his patients would do to live longer and better and included "attend worship every week" alongside the more standard pieces of advice like exercise, drinking water, and eating vegetables. Research has confirmed that prayer has documentable and verifiable benefits in improving one's chances of combating illness. More recently, meditation has been touted as the cure-all for everything from depression to psoriasis. Now the medical community is starting to list practical reasons why one might want to be a regular participant in a faith community. But the benefits are found in attending *regularly*. Every week. Once a month doesn't cut it, not surprisingly. Once a month of eating properly or exercising is unlikely to make much difference either.

Those who are regularly a part of a faith community show less incidence of depression, greater chance of recovery from serious illness, more stable family relationships, and children who are less likely to become drug users.[1] These stats are referenced occasionally by the media, with the adamant explanation that this isn't *religious* advice. "It's because people are less isolated" comes the caveat. It isn't *faith* that is important, but the actions that make a difference.

---

1. Brian Bethune and Genna Buck, "The Science Is In: God Is the Answer," *Maclean's Magazine*, March 30, 2015, *https://www.macleans.ca/society/science/god-is-the-answer/*.

Religion-without-belief is seen as a way of addressing our individual need to live longer and better lives.

At the heart of our Christian faith is a Lord who never seemed to mind that people came to him because they needed something. He rather expected that need might be the starting line of faith.

Right Relationship

In poet Mary Karr's memoir *Lit*, she describes her journey to sobriety, and in the process, her journey into a life of faith. She kicked and screamed every step of the way. When she found herself in rehab once again, a mentor addressed her need with spiritual advice:

> "You have to start giving the higher-power thing a try—it's the only suggestion you skirted. You didn't pray."
>
> Jenny doesn't pray, I say, and she's been sober twenty years.
>
> And Jenny's disposition?
>
> Mean as a snake, I confirm.
>
> "You may find sober people who don't pray, but all the happy ones have some kind of regular meditative or spiritual practice."[2]

AA mandates for alcoholics to be part of a group and to acknowledge a higher power in order to attain healing. Likewise, one way or the other, the Living Diet requires a commitment to other- *and* Other-centeredness. We cannot eat in a way that honors our body and the food we eat as the gifts they are, we cannot discover the blessing of our physical lives, the taste and flavor and pleasure built into this simple act of survival, if we act as if we are alone.

Give Us Today . . .

The most famous prayer of the Christian faith was a response Jesus offered to his disciples when they asked him how to pray. Any of us who were brought up in church can rattle off the Lord's Prayer without a second thought, along with a good number of non-Christians who

---

2. Mary Karr, *Lit* (New York: HarperCollins, 2009), 217.

managed to pick up this prayer by osmosis through a culture still in so many ways permeated with Christian language. Although it is a text I have studied and on which I have meditated, it was only recently that I noticed something of enormous importance about the prayer.

"Lord, teach us to pray," Jesus's followers asked. And after the introductory address to our Sovereign God, Jesus taught his disciples to phrase every petition, not for their individual selves, but for Us. *Give **us** today our daily bread.*

At the center of the Christian faith is a communal prayer that in one simple sentence outlines what right relationship with food might be by asking that the right relationship be granted. Not to me. But to us.

Give Us

Your will be done on earth as in heaven. Jesus frames our request for food with this opening petition: may our world be refashioned according to what God wants for us. May a new world be made visible.

*Give us today **our daily bread**.* He then goes on to ask that the first thing in this new world is that our relationship with food be made right:

- A world where we come to know divine love with full bellies.
- A world where we are able to identify what we need to live. Receiving this provision draws us closer to God.
- A world where we recognize that we are not individuals, but community. We cannot accurately define our individual needs without also identifying and then seeking to address the needs of those around us.
- A world in which we honor God's name, recognizing our place in the universe, assuming the posture of surrender before the One who created us, which leads us to feed those to whom we are connected.

Jesus made it clear that physical feeding is inextricably tied to emotional and spiritual feeding as well. In God's new kingdom, our bodies signal what we need. Our need binds us together and opens us to receiving food that nourishes, sustains, and brings joy.

A Spiritual Problem

> What do men and women want? Everything! The hunger within us is so deep and powerful that, acknowledged or not, only God is sufficient food.
>
> —John Welch, *Seasons of the Heart*

In an interview, author Lionel Shriver attempted to define the root causes of both overeating and overdieting while avoiding the use of explicitly spiritual language. "We are often driven to eat to feed other hungers . . . that food actually can't meet. And it's hard to say what those hungers are: sometimes they're very vague and free floating, but perhaps we're lonely, not feeling sufficiently loved." In another part of the interview, she comments, "Food is the *idea* of satisfaction, rather than satisfaction itself. That is what makes it so powerful. When we're feeling that aimless need for something and we can't put our finger on it, half the time we're just going to reach for a biscuit."[3]

I don't know what Shriver's relationship with organized religion has been. I know that, through experience or through reputation, many have developed a distrust of faith language. Shriver might distrust organized religion. Or she might worry that others will distrust her if she were to show her hand with anything too spiritual in a public broadcasting interview.

As the author of this book, I run a different sort of risk. You, the reader, expect me to speak from a religious point of view. You will not have been surprised that I have done so throughout. While Shriver might say that we are driven to eat to feed "other hungers," I can claim that those hungers are spiritual. However, when I come to this part of the Living Diet, it may be easy to dismiss the practices I am describing as self-serving. I am the pastor of a church congregation. My livelihood depends on people believing that participating in the life of a church is valuable. Whether or not you want to take my word, I nonetheless find it of critical importance to clarify something. I am the pastor of a church congregation because my life has been changed by being part of a church community in ways that I rank as being of ultimate

---

3. Interview with Lionel Shriver on CBC Radio *Q*, Thursday, May 30, 2013.

importance to who I am and who I want to continue to become. I don't want people to belong to a church because I'm a pastor. Rather, I am a pastor because of the difference that belonging to a church has made for me.

And having said that, I share with you the next piece of the Living Diet.

The Living Diet

Worshipping

It doesn't have to be a Christian community. If you are a faithful Jew or Muslim or Buddhist, you should continue to practice faithfully. Not all Christians believe that when Jesus says "I am the way, the truth, and the life" that this means that other religions which have consistently born the fruits of peace and joy and compassion and love are on the wrong path simply because they don't refer to Jesus in doing so. However, for those seeking, or for those whose background is Christian but you have fallen away from practicing the faith, I do invite you to reacquaint yourself with the God who reaches out to us in a human person. I encourage you to rekindle a relationship with Jesus.

Choose a Community

Church shopping has been trendy for many years. People browse the various offerings that meet their criteria: narrow the list of denominations they might consider, check out the preaching, find out if the church programming meets their needs. I know people who have church shopped prayerfully and faithfully and have found a community where they have been able to put down nourishing and long-lasting roots. I also know that approaching church as just one more consumer choice can lead to faith communities that become focused, not on the life and sacrifice and resurrection revealed in Jesus, but to meeting a wide variety of individual consumer preferences.

Here are some other guidelines to consider in finding a worshipping community:

1. **Go Local.** I have extolled the benefits of local eating. The same logic bears on local worshipping. The days seem to have long since passed when churches were populated by their parish—the people who lived within a certain radius of the physical church building. Most people drive to church, and many pass several other church options on their way to their destination. The Living Diet seeks to reconnect our bodies with a sense of physical relationship and therefore responsibility and blessing for the world around us. Participating in a congregation that is in our own neighborhood opens a number of possibilities. We can walk or bike to worship, deepening our understanding of the people who live around us, the needs and the graces surrounding us. Going local allows us to let go, for a moment, of choosing, and instead to allow ourselves to be chosen. We are chosen by virtue of where we are. And therefore, by virtue of where we are, we have something both to give, and to receive.

2. **Where Can I Be of Service?** President John F. Kennedy said, "Ask not what my country can do for me, but what I can do for my country." It is a well-known quote, but his words run deeply contrary to how most of us live most of the time. We are so busy trying to meet our own needs, to find the right alignment of preferences that allow us to feel like we have arrived somewhere, that we miss the more important question of where we can have something to offer. So much of the dissatisfaction in our churches, not to mention our lives, stems from our disappointment that the place doesn't measure up: the people are too gossipy and narrow-minded, the Sunday school is too small, the service is too long, the preaching is too uncomfortable, the beliefs are too loose or too strict.

   I have a friend who believes she is called to be a priest. She is Roman Catholic. And when I asked her why she continues to be Roman Catholic when she can't be a priest, her answer is, "I have to stay in order to be part of how things will change." It is a faithful and surprising outlook. And while I'm not sure I could be so patient, I admire her for it.

   Don't look for the church that match.com would select for you if it were into church dating. Look for the church where something is being asked of you.

3.   **The First Ten Minutes.** This might not sound like much of a sales pitch on joining a church, but bear with me. I talked about this in the section on MOVING. There is a lesson in here, too, about worship.

In many situations, the first ten minutes are the worst. When I am out jogging, I feel most discouraged, out of breath, and negative in the first ten minutes. I dread how long I still have to run; I psych myself out, believing that I don't have it in me to make it through; I am conscious of every struggling breath, every twinge in my side, every ache in my knees. But if I can just get through those first ten minutes, I begin to forget. I get into a rhythm. Adrenaline kicks in. I begin to focus on something other than myself.

We can look for the quick-fix version of church, just like we can look for the quick-fix version of diets. We can look for the church that will entertain and stimulate and impress. Does it sound like I'm criticizing churches that use popular music, hot coffee, and catchy sermon topics to hook people? I'm not. I have been part of leading church communities that have experimented with all of those things, often with success in reaching new people. But, whether we are wowed right away or whether we end up in a place with music and rituals that feel uncomfortable and unfamiliar, worship is like those first ten minutes of running. It might feel like a long and uncertain path. We might think we can't breathe well or find a rhythm. We might conclude we're really not cut out for it. We will be able to name very long lists of things that we would rather be doing. Nobody will think anything less of us if we stay in bed and then go to brunch. Remember, the first ten minutes are the worst. If we can stick with it, we begin to forget ourselves and find a rhythm that makes our hearts sing.

Learn from Church

Here are some of the ways worship can help us learn to eat better and feel better about our bodies.

Gratitude. The service of communion is often called Eucharist, which means *thanksgiving*. Christian worship begins and ends with opening our eyes to receive the blessings before us, to see in the ordinary elements of bread, wine, and people, the extraordinary work of God present and alive in our world, claiming us, all of us, all of creation, as holy.

Generosity. Out of gratitude comes generosity. When we truly see what we have received, we also become able to see what we have to give.

Prayer. The act of prayer is varied and constantly evolving: conversation, connection, honest reflection of who we are, and listening for who we are to welcome and include. Prayer is receiving, abiding, beholding, and being held. Although it is where we get to be most real in our lives, a shocking number of us feel inept as people of prayer, uncomfortable with doing it or speaking of it, often apathetic about carving out any sort of space for allowing prayer to shape our lives, believing the lie that prayer is for a particular sort of holy person who has the time or know-how. My friend Kim once pushed back against the idea that there are people who are "good" at prayer, while the rest of us just struggle along. "Nobody can be better at praying *my* prayer than *me*," she said.

The life of worship teaches us to pray. Through silence and music and fellowship and gathering and sending and eating and wondering and listening and speaking and hearing our world brought into the story of Jesus and back out again, we learn in countless different ways what it looks like to pray and that, in fact, prayer is for all of us.

Relationship. I baptized a thirty-year-old parishioner a few years ago. Shortly after his baptism, he came to me railing against the appalling inability of some of his fellow parishioners to articulate their saving relationship with Jesus.

"Welcome to the body of Christ," I told him.

Being part of a faith community is sure to be disappointing at times. People will express their beliefs in strange and even unpalatable ways. Most churches have a problem with gossip. Some parishioners will have conflicting opinions about where and when we should bow in worship and whether or not little boys should be allowed to wear hats in the sanctuary. But through the grace of God, a faith community can also provide a rock-solid experience of strength and support for those in grief, brokenness, or crisis. When we rise to the challenge of working through our quirks with one another to grow closer to God, or commit to praying for one another's needs and joys, or discover a foundation of prayer on which we can rest in our own time of need, we relearn this truth: *We are not alone.* While it can be comforting to be surrounded by the ties of blood or by the bonds of friendships we have chosen, it is even more remarkable, and a greater testament to the truly relational nature of our biology and our existence in the world, to learn to walk with the people who become our siblings through the seemingly arbitrary bond of faith.

Service. The most important thing about worship, other than getting there, is leaving. We gather so we can be sent. We are fed so we can feed others. I have said that Jesus is the one who embodies right relationship with hunger. If that is true, then the church is the community committed to remaining acquainted with hunger, being honest about it and where we believe it leads us. Our worship teaches us to be honest about our own needs so that we can then be of service to the needs of our world.

Gratitude, generosity, prayer, relationship and service are five practices that rarely, if ever, make it into diet books. And yet, more than counting carbs, bulking up on proteins, or going gluten-free, the things taught to us by worship will change how we see what our bodies, and what we put into our bodies, are for.

Check Your Motives

Isn't there something very wrong about joining a church to feel better about what I eat? Isn't my desperation about my waist size exactly the kind of motive for coming to church that might inspire God to strike me down with lightning? As Jesus made clear time and time again, God doesn't mind people showing up out of desperation. And God knows that we can be a little self-serving, even when it looks like we're doing the right things. Don't worry about coming to church for the wrong reasons. You'll be in good company.

But do take note. Note how these new worshipping practices begin to shape you. Give it time. Like diet and exercise, the more effective changes in life take longer. What, over time, begins to shift in your perspective, in your self-understanding, in your habits and practices outside of church, in your relationships, as you take on this regular discipline of joining a community of faith?

Pray

I wouldn't have thought it to be on God's priority list to care about my privileged twenty-something self, miserably obsessing about how I shouldn't have eaten that extra cinnamon bun. But when Jesus was asked by his followers how to pray, his words were piercingly simple: *give us today our daily bread.*

Don't hesitate to ask for exactly what you need. Lay it down before God—again and again, if need be. The only caveat? *Pray for what others need too.* And while you're at it, notice whether your prayer, over time, begins to change. Because as I pray for *my* daily needs to be met, God is already beginning to work in and through me to understand how my needs are connected to the world around me, how what *we* truly need is actually leading *us* to find and receive life.

chapter
18

Clay Jars

"I Can See the Judgment in Your Eye"

I practice joyful eating in my life, but I still have one major hang-up about food, eating, and bodies: my husband. I worry about what he eats. I am consumed with thoughts about how his eating choices affect his cholesterol, heart, and blood pressure. I irritate him with my worry, and all I can assure him is that my worry comes out of love. I want to grow old with him.

Occasionally my worry explodes into words. "Are you going to eat a potato with all that cheese?" I say it in a lighthearted voice, imagining myself as funny. Dan never finds it funny. Most of the time, I say nothing, which doesn't make it any better.

"You're judging me!" Dan says.

"I didn't say anything," I protest.

"I can see the judgment in your eye," he fires back.

I claim he is wrong, that he's reading his own insecurities onto me. He eats whatever he was planning to eat, and we move on with our lives.

But he is right. There is something else going on in my worry, some place the worry goes to claim a small modicum of power. I am self-righteous, and I am judging him. Deep down, I judge his food choices against my own and I feel, not just concern for his well-being, but also smugness because I believe I make better choices.

Cleaning House

There is a parable that Jesus tells that seems very strange. It certainly doesn't sound like it is describing anything that could be called "Good News."

> "When the unclean spirit has gone out of a person, it wanders through waterless regions looking for a resting place, but not finding any, it says, 'I will return to my house from which I came.' When it comes, it finds it swept and put in order. Then it goes and brings seven other spirits more evil than itself, and they enter and live there; and the last state of that person is worse than the first." (Luke 11:24–26)

Well, there is some good news—a clear warning against dusting, which accounts for my lack of house-cleaning skills.

Okay, I'm kidding.

I have had times when I have been able to be my healthiest self. I eat well. I exercise regularly. I say "no" to desserts, I cut wine out of my life. I begin to feel confident in my own wellness, and I share that confidence with evangelical zeal. I say horribly annoying things like, "I wouldn't know what to do with myself if I had any more energy!" and "kale is my favorite!" and "I bounce out of bed in the morning without even having to set an alarm!" And perhaps feeling well is good, and as far as annoying goes it could be a lot worse. But as a stable place on which to base our lives and our choices, confidence in our own self and our own health and good choices can, in fact, be a very flimsy place indeed.

There is a certain religiosity around the current practices of "clean eating." Judgmentalism can easily become the outward face of choices that an individual makes for health and well-being. As organized religion has declined in North America, healthy eating, and even an obsession around food, has been on the incline. Ironically, "the same things that people rejected in organized religion—self-righteousness, rigid rules, a creeping sort of legalism, and a blind and oftentimes misinformed clinging to its teachings—are again being taken up with zeal in the clean and ethical food movements."[1]

---

1. Sarah Boesveld, "The New Religion: How the Emphasis on 'Clean Eating' Has Created a Moral Hierarchy for Food," *National Post*, Saturday, May 30. 2015.

I have succumbed too many times to the temptation of being religiously self-righteous about my own eating, as well as judgmental of the choices of others. As I cast a holier-than-thou eye at others, I am hard to endure. When I inevitably fall off the bandwagon of rigorous clean living, I am embarrassed.

Jesus's parable is asking *me* to identify something about *myself*. And in case you thought otherwise, it is asking *you* to identify something about *yourself* as well. The good choices that sweep clean the house can cause us to stumble. It is not just destructive to make our lives about mess and carelessness. It is also destructive to come to believe that our lives are saved by our own cleanliness.

The Living Diet: Potentially Risky

There are two serious risks to the Living Diet. It is critical to identify these two risks and that any person seeking to follow these teachings in pursuit of health and wellness be clear about these risks and regularly check their attitudes and practices against them. These risks are all the more fierce because of how seductively and subtly they can wend their way into our thoughts and actions.

The first risk is *paralysis*. It would be easy to read this book and to believe that this is all too demanding and it is impossible to sort out into actual changed behavior and there is no starting point, and how could one person keep track of all of these rules and practices and suggestions anyway? I have been intentional about building freedom and flexibility into the Living Diet; it is not a rule book to be followed, but rather an articulation of the patterns that emerge from our stories and the wisdom passed down through generations. Many of us prefer a rigorous set of rules, though, even if those rules set us up for failure.

It is easy, in the face of potential transformation and freedom, to choose any set of destructive patterns simply because they are familiar, and therefore don't demand too much. It is easy to miss the gentle invitation at the heart of Jesus's way, to hear his words "follow me" as an overwhelming demand rather than a simple call; take one step and see. "Give us today our daily bread. Forgive our debts. Guard us from evil." The Lord's Prayer is essentially the "one step" prayer. Protect us and provide for us right now. Then give us the next step. The other key contained in the Lord's Prayer is "us" and "our." If we keep the next step of those around us in prayer, our next step is easier as well.

The second risk to the Living Diet is *self-righteousness*. Some of the possibilities and changes I have suggested are similar to those made by the secular health and wellness culture. Others have deep spiritual roots. In either case, we can derail ourselves with smugness. When we compare the cleanliness of our houses with others, we run the risk of making a bigger mess. Or of simply being intolerable. Think back to my recurring argument with my husband, Dan. He knows me well. He can read into my innermost heart.

"You're judging me," he says. Deep down, I am. I assess his food choices and I assess my own, and I find his lacking. I am smug and I am self-righteous.

Food and Death

The flip side of my self-righteousness is my own insecurity around food and my body. Yes, it is true that I feel grateful for the food I eat, the exercise I get, and the health of my body. Yes, I have received remarkable healing in my relationship with food and my body. And yes, I have learned to lean on some of the practices of the Living Diet, which keep me well and centered.

And deep down, of course, is the flimsiness of it all. Whatever insight I have gained is carried in a body that doesn't understand everything, makes mistakes, and won't live forever. I can be well and healthy and happy. And there are things about the relationship between the food I eat and the way that my body feels that are still mysterious. My body might, and in fact, will, one day let me down. I might twist an ankle while running; then where would I be without movement? My brain might wear smooth and thin and rob me of the core identity associated with my words and memories. I can eat carefully and cancer cells can still steal in and take command. One day I will inhale and it will be my last breath. None of us gets to usurp our own mortality. Somehow my food and my food choices and my weight and my resolve (or lack of resolve) are all wound up in this truth and mystery.

A healthy relationship with my body and my body's relationship with the world around it requires thought, discernment, gratitude, and surrender. Such life-giving freedom becomes more possible with prayer and with corporate worship in a faith community. But often it is easier to cast the eye of judgment than to enter into the silence and mystery and listening. Human beings are great at tripping ourselves up with religiosity and missing the Spirit. We turn the journey of faith into an institution of rules and regulations that draws clear lines around who is in and who is out. Likewise, we turn our relationship with food and our bodies into numbers and categories, into labels and failures, into a sword of judgment to wield against those who aren't in the fold and a blanket of smugness and self-righteousness for those who are. We have come full circle to the start of this Living Diet journey: our problem with food is a spiritual one.

And to be well spiritually is to be prepared to die.

Remember the Ashes

Within all of the choices about what we eat and how we move, all of the different ways we find of honoring our bodies and living out our relational truth, all of our capacity for ignoring who we are and living in forgetfulness, is the truth that marks all of us—the ones who skate along the surface of life; the ones who try to go deep; the ones who give their lives to newer, better, faster, more; the ones who remember that there is another story that claims us; the ones who don't know where to start; the ones who fool themselves into thinking they have arrived.

Once a year in the Christian pattern of worship, we are gathered by the sign of our mortality. Ash Wednesday is a tough sell to even my most loyal congregants. Whereas the star of Mardi Gras is on the rise—mainstream culture is firmly comfortable with joining in the excuse for debauchery and indulgence—Ash Wednesday's focus on repentance and fasting and death has come to be seen as inaccessible to any but the most pious. This is deeply unfortunate, because of all of the Christian year, Ash Wednesday is the most honest, the most grounded in the experience of, not just the religious, but all of us.

You are dust, and to dust you shall return. The ashes are marked on our foreheads with these haunting and hopeful words. They are spoken to both the ones who are drawing in on their final days and the ones who look to be in the first bloom of life's promise. First and finally, our lives are in the hands of our Creator. For whatever period of time we are granted the gift of the breath of life, we can choose to live as if our beginning and ending matters; we can choose whether to live for ourselves or to live as if our lives are from and for Someone.

Lest we think those choices are too hard to make, the ashes remind us that we start with today. What I do with my life today matters.

Lest we get tricked into believing that our choices are better than someone else's, the ashes teach us humility and surrender.

If we are willing to listen and to be quiet and to pray with others, we can discover in the Christian narrative and Christian worship a stark honesty about death. The way of Jesus teaches us to take up our cross and prepare to die. It turns out that we have to be ready to die in order to be able to learn how to live.

The Living Diet

Dying

The last piece of the Living Diet gives three simple practices for keeping death before us. Death might seem like the least obvious way of embracing a positive relationship with food and bodies, and yet it can allow the most powerful corrective to the risks of the Living Diet. To choose to embrace our mortality is also to embrace the choices we can make today and to surrender to the choices that are not ours to make. And to choose and to surrender is ultimately to turn toward hope and away from fear. It is to be pulled back, or set free, from falling over either the brink of paralysis or the brink of smugness.

It is worth noting that, in fact, death will liberate you from both of these things anyway. One day you will die and you will no longer be overwhelmed by the choices that are yours in this life to make. One day you will die and you will no longer cast your eye of judgment on the choices anyone else is making.

You can wait to be set free. Or you can choose now. Then you can choose again tomorrow. And the day after that. You can keep

Continued

The Living Diet *Continued*

choosing as you keep remembering that one day you will die. And because one day you will die, you can make the choices that give you life today. You can look with compassion on the choices that the people to whom you are related are making. Choose honesty about your mortality and therefore choose living life.

1. Speak about Your Death

You will need to practice. Practice around people who are safe. Practice speaking about your own death and not turning your words into either a joke or a threat; clear your overtones of anything that sounds like silliness or suicide. It might take time for your words to not feel loaded and fearful. You will have no control over how your words will be received, but practice speaking with honesty and hopefulness. Practice is good. Practice naming the truth that one day you will die. Practice articulating the choices you would like to make about your inevitable death in the midst of the choices that will not be yours.

2. Communal Prayer

Any Christian worship worth its salt makes reference to the mortal reality of our nature and the intimately connected cycles of death and life. To participate regularly in the set pattern of the Christian tradition is to enter into the ashes and the rebirth, into the burning and drowning, and into the renewal and exodus—to walk to the cross and to be raised at the dawn of the new morning. To be part of a community's prayer is to be intimately connected to the hope and freedom of the life we are given and that one day will end.

3. Keep Track of the Saints

Death is feared in our culture. This fear is no doubt connected to the denial and sterilization in which we wrap our food up as products to be consumed rather than as the relationship of life in which we live. The move toward doctor-assisted death is a relief to many, an antidote to the possibility of suffering, and more importantly, to the powerlessness that we have come to see as a stripping of our individual dignity.

"If I ever get like that," I have heard loved ones say, "just take me out to a field somewhere and shoot me." As more of us face dementia at the end of our lives, a deep-seated fear of loss of control tightens its grip and buries itself deeper into our collective consciousness. We have done little to talk about how this fear shapes the values and practices we share.

I participated in a funeral a few years ago for one of our generation's leading mathematicians who eventually was diagnosed with Alzheimer's. He couldn't choose to keep his memories, but he actively chose to find his own changing brain patterns fascinating; he wrote and reflected on the process of losing his own mind and shared his thoughts with his loved ones. I am inspired by his example. I know that I may one day succumb to dementia. I pray that, should this happen, I will simply find the grace to choose curiosity over embarrassment.

Keep track of those who die well, lest we come to believe that dying well is merely a stroke of luck, or that passing from this life to the next without pain is normal. Acquaint yourselves with the experiences of those who suffer and still die with love and light around them. Keep track of the choices that can be made within the circumstances that are not of our choosing. Keep track of the saints: not the perfect ones, but the ones who show us something of how we would like to live. And how to die.

We Have This Treasure in Clay Jars (2 Cor. 4:7)

I opened my Thanksgiving letter one year to my congregation with these words:

> I write this letter on the heels of having spent my day off with my grandmother. She is ninety-one. She went out to work as a young preteen girl in the Depression; she sent a fiancé off to fight in the Second World War, buried a child, has been widowed twice, and is in the process now of transitioning into long-term care. Throughout

those challenges and tragedies, she has moved with a graciousness and lightness that has led me to name her as one of the most important influences in my life. She isn't weighed down with fear and regret, she is able to accept what is, and more than that, to recognize blessings and give thanks.

One of the great writers and evangelists of the church, Paul, wrote some of his most powerful passages from prison. He was seen as a direct threat to the sovereignty of Caesar because of his fiery counter-proclamation, "Jesus is Lord." As he awaited execution, he was able to hold up the fragility of his own life as good:

> For it is the God who said, "Let light shine out of darkness," who has shone in our hearts to give the light of the knowledge of the glory of God in the face of Jesus Christ. But we have this treasure in clay jars, so that it may be made clear that this extraordinary power belongs to God and does not come from us. We are afflicted in every way, but not crushed; perplexed, but not driven to despair; persecuted, but not forsaken; struck down, but not destroyed; always carrying in the body the death of Jesus, so that the life of Jesus may also be made visible in our bodies. For while we live, we are always being given up to death for Jesus' sake, so that the life of Jesus may be made visible in our mortal flesh. So death is at work in us, but life in you. (2 Cor. 4:6–12)

We might, here and there, share in something of light and truth. At some point, our clay jars will break or crumble, and that light and truth will no longer be ours to hold. And if we can celebrate that it never was ours, that we were only sharing in something far bigger than ourselves, far bigger than any of us, then we can also celebrate and give thanks for the clay.

My grandmother had been disappearing from us for several years, her appetite dwindling—"food just doesn't taste the same anymore." We encouraged her to eat more and plied her with the sweet things she had craved in more robust days. We worried about her frailty and how her bones were becoming more prominent under her thinning skin.

"Have you ever been with someone who stopped eating?" my friend and spiritual director, Kevin, asked me once. "Whose life ran its natural course and they weren't going to get better so they stopped eating? Have you ever been with them when they died? It's a good death. There is something really ancient and natural about it. In some cultures, an elder would know their time was near and would just walk out into the woods one day and stop eating and not come back." We come into this world crying for food. We eat and therefore we live. And in the completion of a good and full life, when that life is transitioning into something else, how right it can be that the craving and the driving starts to lift, the body's reserves begin to disappear, death becomes a gentle surrender—not to an ending, but to the next chapter.

My grandmother died several months after I wrote that letter. She understood the fragility of life. She did not fear the reality of death and loss. Therefore, she was able to embrace living. She died with my brother, my parents, and me by her side. Graciousness and lightness and gratitude filled her room and filled our hearts as we held her hands and she breathed her last. Those qualities that I noted in her at Thanksgiving—an ability to accept what is, to recognize blessings, and give thanks—culminated in the peace and beauty in which she died.

chapter

19

A Theology of Cake

It is not good to eat much honey, or to seek honor on top of honor.
(Prov. 25:27)

am known for my love of cake. This is because the congregations I
have served have noticed a significant upswing in the amount of cake
they consume when I join them. I can think of all kinds of occasions
that deserve to be celebrated, and few things signal celebration more to
me than an enormous cake that all can share.

I love cake. I love celebrating with cake. I don't care so much
whether or not I eat the cake. It isn't my irresistible temptation. I can
watch a roomful of people munching on slices of chocolate or vanilla
cake without needing to join in. Unless.

Unless the cake is homemade. Unless it is iced with a stiff buttercream icing. Unless the cake is moist and dense—the denser the better.
As much as I like cake, the most appalling dessert, in my opinion, is angel
food cake. What's the point? Any treat whose signature characteristic is
that it is "light" doesn't deserve the title of "dessert." When my mother
makes her buttered almond cake—the recipe from a Mennonite restaurant we used to frequent in the Kitchener-Waterloo area when I was very
young—all bets are off. When Faith, in my current congregation, shows
up with her double-layer chocolate slab cake, the chocolate rich and not
too sweet, the icing thick and creamy and decorated with words of love,
encouragement, celebration, or congratulations (depending on the occasion), I have to restrain myself from elbowing people out of the way.

I will very occasionally carve out an afternoon to make a cake myself. Dan generally dreads and discourages these occasions because of the mess I make and because of the drama that ensues when things inevitably don't go quite according to plan, although he is just as thrilled as everyone else with the finished product. Our family's favorite of my offerings is a three-layer maple cake, stacked with fresh raspberries and the most buttery buttercream imaginable. My cakes tend to look awful. I respect others who master the intricacies of cake decorating, but my care and attention are only concerned with the taste. When I serve one that is particularly sad-looking, I remind people that it has love baked into every morsel. I believe you can taste the love.

✿ ✿ ✿

The first time I ran a half marathon, I thought that a seriously restricted diet would be the key to my racing success. I was particularly religious about a six-week fast from sugar, believing it would clear up my skin, lighten my feet, and fill me with energy. However, as I ran up the first long hill on the exceptionally hilly course, it wasn't my legs that felt sore; I was gripped by an overall exhaustion.

"I could just curl up on the side of the road and take a nap," I told my friend Jeff, a fierce running competitor, who accompanied me through the grueling 21 kilometers as a personal favor. He didn't say anything, but I could feel his respect for me dip. I'm sure that he never once wanted to have a nap while he was racing.

I continued to muse out loud to him about my condition. Running is a spiritual discipline for me, which is why I find it so appealing to have a running companion who is willing to chit-chat. It's a good distraction from the more demanding work of prayer and reflection. "I think I just don't have everything figured out yet with my eating," I suggested. Why, after eating like a celebrity for all of these weeks, was my energy drooping? Where was the lightness I was supposed to feel in my feet? It made me want to shake my fists at the heavens. Surely my sense of entitlement was justified. No pain, no gain. So the reverse should also be true. Pain *equals* gain. I had sacrificed, I should be rewarded.

Jeff said nothing. He raised an eyebrow in a flicker of judgment, which I caught at the time and failed to interpret.

✹ ✹ ✹

Around that same time, I was seeing Gloria, a nutritionist and health guru (mentioned in chapter 11). The kids' school year had started back up, and I was feeling foggy and exhausted. We went through what I had been eating. She tested me on a few different trigger foods. Nothing was answering the question. So, she started probing a little deeper. Was there an anxiety? Something weighing on my mind? I was going through a difficult time with my daughter. She was upset about starting grade one, and she always seemed to be asking more of me than I, as a full-time working parent, was able to give.

"It is good that you work, you know," Gloria told me, responding to the sentiments I was having trouble articulating. "Your work is important and good. And it's okay that you are a working parent." The guilt welled up inside me and began leaking out in a stream of tears. No matter how much I offered, how much time I gave, it was never enough.

We talked more about the feelings of inadequacy and the guilt that I couldn't even imagine living without. It became a counselling session with food and diet slipping off the front burner for the rest of our time together. I prayed about my dilemma. In the following weeks I found that Cecilia and I could go biking together in the evenings—she on her two-wheeler, and me running beside her. As we spent time together doing something that we both loved, our relationship settled and some of my mental fog lifted.

It is surprising how often we fail to identify that our physical and mental and spiritual problems can be caused by our food choices. But, with the same token, sometimes our problems aren't really about food at all.

I now know why I was feeling droopy in that half marathon. It was partly because I wasn't eating enough. As I have continued to run and to train for long distances, I have discovered that if I want to properly fuel myself, I can anticipate putting *on* a little weight. Eating becomes a very different affair when the consequences of not keeping the fuel tank topped up are physical injury and physical burn-out. I was not consuming enough calories while running. I had to learn that fatigue while running is my body's signal that it is hungry. Running is the only time that I don't feel like eating. When I'm in the middle of an especially long distance, I more likely feel like vomiting. But unless I force some replenishing sugars into my system, I feel the same exhaustion that baffled me in that first race.

However, there was an even more important reason for my tired muscles that day. I didn't train enough. Jeff had looked at the half marathon course as soon as I talked about signing up. "It's hilly," he told me. "You'll want to practice your hills." He had helped me map out a training regime, balancing out long slow runs with short faster ones, and mixed in regular timed sprints up some of Orillia's steepest hills. I had not followed his plan. I put in the weekly targets for mileage, but I never got around to his more rigorous suggestions. Not surprisingly, giving up dessert wasn't enough to rocket me over hills for which I had not prepared. Likewise, my mental fogginess several months later was not from cheating with chocolate cake, but because of the deeper anxieties of living up to too many expectations and a lifelong habit of wearing guilt like a mantle.

Although I am as likely to assume this as anyone, *the answer isn't just food.*

Food Is Not . . . Art / Religion / THE Answer

William Deresiewicz wrote what ended up being a controversial article in the *New York Times* in 2012. He noted that food has taken the place of art as the pinnacle of cultural achievement:

> Just as aestheticism, the religion of art, inherited the position of Christianity among the progressive classes around the turn of the 20th century, so has foodism taken over from aestheticism around the turn of the 21st. Now we read the gospel according, not to Joyce or Proust, but to Michael Pollan and Alice Waters. . . . Food now expresses the symbolic values and absorbs the spiritual energies of the educated class. It has become invested

with the meaning of life. It is seen as the path to salvation, for the self and humanity both.[1]

The reaction to his piece did much to cement his argument. The outraged responses indicated that, in fact, art/culture/religion is exactly what food has become to us. While so many Western people struggle with waistlines and healthy eating choices, and at the same time junk food still appears to have almost total domination of our diets, the "foodie" movement obsesses about the intricacies of the taste, texture, age, and origin of our food items, and delights in the blending of ingredients, or the perfect execution of a gourmet dish.

I am not a gourmand or even an amateur weekend chef. I am very keenly aware of how food is tied to spirit, to friendship, to love. But as I was reminded with Jeff and Gloria, food, like anything else, can become an idol: a distraction from engaging with anything deeper than menu choices, a distraction from looking inward and wondering how old habits or laziness-inducing crutches might be challenged.

Trend or Wisdom?

I read the tabloid magazines about once a year, on Boxing Day. We circulate the year-end roundup of trashy offerings around our family and pass comment on the various celebrities. "Who are the Kardashians anyway, and why are they famous?" my mom asks every year. We don't ever have an adequate answer. The level of snarkiness on these pages shocks me out of reading them for the next twelve months. So-called friends dish on their famous acquaintances, beautiful women are lined up side by side and judged according to who wears a particular outfit better, and newly separated former Hollywood power couples are compared to assess who is moving on better, which can apparently be ascertained primarily by deciding whose skin looks better. Toward the back is an inevitable spread of the newest body and wellness trends—everything from bone broth to probiotic waters to organic, gluten-free meal subscription services starting at $100 a pop.

---

1. William Deresiewicz, "A Matter of Taste?" *New York Times*, October 26, 2012.

As ridiculous as these things sound, exotic and strange health trends don't belong only to the Hollywood elite. My various circles of friends regularly wax eloquent on a whole range of food practices that never fail to surprise me: pink salt as seasoning, gargling with coconut oil, the newest gluten-free products, the most innovative replacements for sugar. The stream of health information is forever shifting and expanding.

In our modern-day North American food landscape, we need guidance in how to distinguish wisdom in the midst of trendiness; how to guard against the seductive belief that our food choices serve only us; how to allow ourselves to continue to be open to new learning in the endless mystery of being a body in this world.

Sugar offers a key.

The Battle

I'm not going to offer the key that you are probably expecting. I can testify to the problems sugar causes. My husband and I have a personal battle with sugar as we try to parent our children. I don't need a dietician, dentist, or documentary to explain the effects of sugar. I have experienced the alarming transformation that takes place in my children when they have too much sweet stuff. They become hyper, then angry, then irrational, then mean, hot-tempered, and explosive. As much as I try to control their sugar intake, there are people all around them—not just the grandparents who have earned the right to spoil their grandchildren, but teachers and classmates, soccer parents, hairdressers, waiters—who give out suckers and sweets with a blithe smile, free of any sympathy for, or understanding of, the harm they are causing. That we celebrate with something laden with the white stuff is built into the fabric of society. I can't even begin to count how many times we have ended birthday parties, special family trips and vacations, or Christmas get-togethers with kids screaming and crying because their sugar-addled minds have skimmed over all of the beauty of the day to fixate on one injustice, one grievance, or one frustration. As my husband notes, it's difficult to even justify getting angry with them. We're enablers, or at least complacent, in their consuming an excess of a substance that we know brings them to a place of misery.

From my own times of abstinence, I can fill out the story on sugar's evils. I now notice how even small amounts of dessert affect me, how the cloying sweetness of many of our favorite treats fills my mouth in an unpleasant way, how they give me a buzz of energy and then a crash of fog and dopiness. At times, I have been so convinced by my sugar-free existence that it has been easy to turn down treats because temptation for the stuff has temporarily evaporated. I know that I am a more patient, even-tempered, and productive person without sugar in my life.

Unfortunately, I am also intolerable in other ways. Life *without* sugar also has its problems. While on my high horse, I have made spiritual claims about the benefits of a sweet-free life. After all, I am better able to juggle my responsibilities; my life comes into sharp, clear focus. Sugar-free living allows me to better serve God. The shadow to this focus and energy is that I miss out on the softer, sweeter side of life, the ability to respond to celebrations and opportunities with a gentle bending of the rules, sharing in an indulgence, and appreciating the offering of someone else's time and energy in making a dessert to mark an occasion.

My friend George commented once about the communion wine we used at my previous parish in Orillia. It was a fortified wine, higher on the sugar scale.

"I know it's more sophisticated to drink dry reds," he said, "but it seems right that in the kingdom of God, we should be left with a sweet taste in our mouth."

In the kingdom of God, we should be left with a sweet taste in our mouth. The shadow is in both the sweetness and the abstinence from it. Somehow, in the wisdom of our good Creator, there must be a possibility to have our cake and eat it too. (Why else would you have cake except to eat it?) Abstinence needs to be redeemed by the occasional taste of honey. And mindless consumption needs to be redeemed by recognizing that there is a choice to be reclaimed. In the struggle to serve and the easy pitfalls of indulgence all around us in our privileged existence, there is the offer of God's abundant life.

Powerful Gifts

Abundant life has something to do with the nonstop work of growing up, which at its core involves figuring out how to receive God's good gifts. We have long recognized that sex and alcohol are potent, powerful gifts from God. They are gifts that can be extremely dangerous and destructive if misused. There are those who are called to celibacy because of circumstance or vocation. And in that celibacy, they have to figure out how to celebrate, rather than judge, how others are able to use the gift of sex to bring life and joy. There are those who need to be sober because of the disease of addiction, because for some there is no way to allow any amount of alcohol into their lives without it taking over. And in that sobriety, the alcoholic may eventually learn how to accept the moderate drinking of others.

I wonder how we might come to see sugar in a similar way. The alarm bells are ringing all across the globe calling for a better understanding of the serious harm that our current levels of sugar consumption cause for human health. We need tighter regulations and greater transparency across the food industry in order to help our human family to make healthier choices. This may be right and good. But to label sugar as evil is to read our human misuse of sugar onto sugar itself. In other words, sugar isn't evil. It is a powerful gift. Our mindless use of that powerful gift, or the food industry's deliberate use of that powerful gift to craft low-quality ingredients into temptations too powerful to resist, have damaging consequences.

Moses, Aaron, and Miriam were charged with leading the people of Israel out of slavery and into the freedom of the Promised Land. It took them forty years of wandering through the wilderness to get there, to shed the physical and mental bonds of their former captivity and to begin to conceive of how they might enter into and receive a "land flowing with milk and honey." The history of Israel is the story of God's hand in breaking the bonds of oppression. It can also serve as an archetype for God's invitation to be set free from our privileged forgetfulness, to receive our food, our drink, our freedom, and our life itself as offered by the very hand of God's generous provision. It is the journey into remembering how these gifts are to be used not merely for ourselves, but as expressions of service and gratitude, relationship with God, and responsibility to others. When we are in right relationship with one another and with the world that God made, a generous sweetness opens up to us.

Sweeter than Honey

I am not at my best either when voiding my life of sweets or when my hand is compulsively in the cookie jar. I am not at my best as a parent, a friend, a neighbor, or the stranger in the grocery store when I have swung to either extreme. My observation of others corroborates my own experience. I don't know anybody who perpetually refrains from dessert whom I particularly care to be my companion more than in small doses. Nor do I know anyone enslaved to the addiction of sugar who doesn't yearn for freedom, even while guarding against that yearning through practiced humor or stealthy eating practices.

The witness of our ancestors in faith suggests that these are lessons we must continually learn. God's more powerful gifts require a sort of vigilant thoughtfulness. They can too easily be used to control and exploit, or more typically, with the mindlessness of the well-trained consumer, simply filling my time chasing down one desire after another. Every day we have to navigate, with our children and loved ones, the minefield of Pinocchio's Pleasure Island on which we currently live, where God's invitation to learn to be a grown up has never mattered so much, and where we are literally plied with enough sugar and fun to indulge ourselves to death. Instead, we can learn and relearn how to choose God's abundant life, that finicky recipe of both restraint and indulgence, recognizing our agency in choosing to not have something that we can have, and giving thanks for the sweet gifts we also receive along the way.

In this vigilant thoughtfulness, there is grace. With sugar, as with sex and alcohol, there are moments where we can receive goodness—saying "yes" is uncomplicated, and it is an unqualified good. Cake is the dessert for which I am known. But I am going to end with a story that features another dessert.

Cherry Pie

Every December my dad and I carve out a Sunday afternoon for baking. We solve the worries of the world as we mix the ingredients, roll the dough, add the teeming cup of sugar to the frozen cherries and form the pie. My favorite part comes in poking the holes in the crust, lightly carving an awkward "C" on the top, and brushing the pie with the heavy cream that sits in my fridge because it is holiday time, and holidays call for heavy cream. I dust the pie with sugar and my dad puts it in the oven.

There are no questions of abstinence or indulgence, or sugar-induced bad moods, or whether the kids have already had too much sweet stuff when that fresh pie is sliced and served at our supper table.

The pie dissolves our food idols in that moment. There is no way to taste the buttery fresh-out-of-the-oven pastry and sweet, tart cherries and not know that the experience points us far beyond diets and foodie culture and proper calorie intake to a gift of God, manifested in community, story, and, perhaps above all, flavor.

The only thing to do is to eat it together with joy.

Acknowledgments

Around the time that my husband, Dan, and I might have considered having a third child, we instead each embarked on another sort of creative venture. He began work on his doctorate and I began writing this book. Both projects came to fruition within a week of one another: Dan successfully defending his thesis and me hearing from Milton Brasher-Cunningham at Church Publishing that he would be my editor on my soon-to-be-published book. This book is "my third baby." I am so grateful that Dan and I have been able to make room for these life-giving pieces of creativity in the shape of our family's life together. And that gratitude now extends to Milton in being such an ideal partner—a "kindred stomach"—in getting this book ready for publication.

Prior to Milton, I had three extraordinarily generous friends edit my manuscript in its earlier iterations. Thank you Pauline Horton, Ursula Irwin, and Catherine Pate.

I am grateful, too, to the various readers who have offered encouragement, insight, and suggestions along the way: Kevin Block, Kevin Flynn, Lindsey Hoover, Phil Jackman, Jay Koyle, Tanya Kuzmanovic, Mike Ripmeester, and Pam Szegvary. The turning point for me in understanding what I was writing and why it mattered, and then finding a publisher for this book, was attending the Collegeville Institute in Minnesota in 2017. Big thanks go out to the institute for creating such a beautiful space to nurture theological writing, to our workshop leaders Thomas G. Long and Sari Fordham for their support and wisdom that made us all better writers, thank you to that whole cohort and especially my roommate, Bromleigh McCleneghan, for ideas, connections, and friendship.

I dedicated this book to St. David's in Orillia and St. George's in St. Catharines, the two communities in which I served as I was writing this book. They have both taught me—as they gather around God's table, join in fellowship together, and feed the hungry—what joyful eating is and how it can change people, neighborhoods, and worlds.

I wrote this book for them. But I also wrote this book because of my family. Thank you to my parents, John and Susan, for making home cooking, extravagant feasting, and open table fellowship central to our family's life. Thank you to my grandparents, Gordon, Jean, Elma, Bill, and Bill, for creating such powerful patterns of food and faith in our lives, and thank you especially to my two grandmothers for passing along strength and love and fantastic recipes. Thank you to Dan's parents, Helen and Glen, both gone too soon, but the imprint of their love rests always on our family. And Helen's melt-in-your-mouth cabbage rolls were the best the world has ever known.

As I said at the outset, I am profoundly grateful now as I raise my own family that Dan has embraced with me a home life that centers around the great blessings of faith and food. To my children, Cecilia and Gordon, it is an astonishing thing to watch you grow into all of your own creative and generous pursuits. I give thanks every day for the traditions we continue together, for the new patterns of flavor and love and joy we now embrace.